ANSWERS IN GLAUCOMA

ANSWERS IN GLAUCOMA

REMO SUSANNA JR.

- Associate Professor, University of São Paulo, Brazil
- Director and Chief, Glaucoma Service University of São Paulo, Brazil

ROBERT N. WEINREB

- Professor of Ophthalmology
- Director, Hamilton Glaucoma Center University of California San Diego, USA

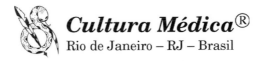
Cultura Médica®
Rio de Janeiro – RJ – Brasil

CIP-BRAZIL. CATALOGAÇÃO-NA-FONTE
SINDICATO NACIONAL DOS EDITORES DE LIVROS, RJ, BRAZIL

S962g

Susanna Junior, Remo
    Glaucoma : Answers in Glaucoma / Remo Susanna Jr.,
Robert N. Weinreb. – Rio de Janeiro, Brazil : Cultura Médica, 2005
    336p. : il. ;

    Includes Bibliographical references and index.
    ISBN 85-7006-357-1

    1. Glaucoma.   I. Weinreb, Robert N., 1949. II. Title.

05-0008

CDD 617.741
CDU 617.7–0007.681

© Copyright 2005, by *Cultura Médica*®

Printed in Brazil

Edition in Portuguese, 2005
Edition in Espanish, 2005

Cultura Médica®

Rua São Francisco Xavier, 111
20550-010 – Rio de Janeiro – RJ – Brazil
Tel.: 55-21-2567-3888 – Fax: 55-21-2569-5443
site: www.culturamedica.com.br
e-mail: cultura@culturamedica.com.br

Contributors

Ahmad A. Aref, BS

- University Eye Specialists Chicago Center for Vision Research and the Department of Ophthalmology, Northwestern University Chicago, Illinois, USA

Anders Heijl, MD, PhD

- Professor and Chairman, Department of Ophthalmology, Malmö University Hospital Malmö, Sweden

Andrew C. Crichton, MD

- Clinical Associate Professor Departament of Ophthalmology, University of Calgary, Alberta, Canada

Anita S. Y. Chan, MRCS(Ed), M.Med

- Singapore National Eye Center, Singapore

Balwantray C. Chauhan, PhD

- Professor and Research Director Department of Ophthalmology Dalhousie University of Halifax, Nova Scotia, Canada

Catherine Boden, PhD

- Assistant Research Scientist, Visual Function Laboratory, Hamilton Glaucoma Center, University of California at San Diego, La Jolla, California, USA

Celso Tello, MD

- Assistant Professor of Ophthalmology, Associate Director, Glaucoma Service The New York Eye and Ear Infirmary, New York, USA

Christopher A. Girkin, MD

- Associate Professor Director Glaucoma Service, Department of Ophthalmology, School of Medicine, University of Alabama, Birmingham, USA

Claude F. Burgoyne, MD

- LSU Eye Center, Louisiana State University Health Sciences Center, New Orleans and the Department of Biomedical Engineering, Tulane University, New Orleans, USA

Clive Migdal, MD, FRCS, FRCOphth

- Clinical Director and Charman of Ophthalmology Departament Western Eye Hospital, London United Kingdom, England

Curt Hartleben, MD

- Head Clinical Research in Glaucoma, Instituto de Oftalmologia Conde Valenciana Mexico City, Mexico

Dale K. Heuer, MD

- Professor and Chairman, Department of Ophthalmology, Medical College of Wisconsin, Milwaukee, USA

Daniel Grigera, MD

- Head, Glaucoma Service, Hospital Oftalmológico Santa Lucia, Buenos Aires, Argentina. Assistant Professor of Ophthalmology, Universidad del Salvador, Buenos Aires, Argentina

Don Minckler, MD

- Professor & Director of Glaucoma Services, Doheny Eye Institute, University of Southern California, Keck School of Medicine, Los Angeles, USA

Douglas H. Johnson, MD

- Professor of Ophthalmology, Mayo Clinic, College of Medicine, Rochester, Minnesota, USA

Douglas R. Anderson, MD

- Professor of Ophthalmology and Douglas R. Anderson Chair in Ophthalmology, Bascom Palmer Eye Institute, Department of Ophthalmology, University of Miami School of Medicine, Miami, USA

Erik L. Greve, MD

- Emeritus Professor the Glaucoma Department University of Amsterdam, the Netherlands
- Executive Vice-President, Association of International Glaucoma Societies
- Chief and Managing Editor of International Glaucoma Review

Felipe A. Medeiros, MD

- Assistant Clinical Professor, Hamilton Glaucoma Center and Department of Ophthalmology, University of California San Diego, USA

Felix Gil Carrasco, MD

- Professor Glaucoma Service Universidad Nacional Autonoma de Mexico, Mexico City, Mexico

George A. Cioffi, MD

- Director of Glaucoma Service Devers Eye Institute, Portland, Oregon, USA

Henry Jampel, MD, MHS

- Associate Professor of Ophthalmology, Wilmer Eye Institute, Johns Hopkins University, USA

Heryberto S. Alvim, MD

- Research Fellow, Glaucoma Service, Wills Eye Hospital/Jefferson Medical College, Philadelphia, Pennsylvania. Cpontifícia Universidade Católica de São Paulo, Sorocaba, SP, Brasil

Ivan Goldberg, MB. BS, FRACO

- Director Glaucoma Service, Eye Associates and Sydney Eye Hospital Sydney, Australia

James D. Brandt, MD

- Professor of Ophthalmology & Director, Glaucoma Service University of California, USA

Jeffrey M. Liebmann, MD

- Clinical Professor of Ophthalmology, New York University School of Medicine Director, Glaucoma Services, Manhattan Eye, Ear, & Throat Hospital, New York University Medical Center, New York City, USA

Jody Piltz-Seymour, MD

- Associate Professor, University of Pennsylvania School of Medicine, Director Glaucoma Service, Scheie Eye Institute, USA

Joel S. Schuman, MD, UPMC

- Eye and Ear Foundation Professor and Chairman of Ophthalmology, University of Pittsburgh School of Medicine and Director of the University of Pittsburgh Medical Center, Eye Center, Pittsburgh, USA

Jonathan G. Crowston PhD, MD

- Assistant Clinical Professor, Hamilton Glaucoma Center, University California, San Diego, California, USA

Jost B. Jonas, MD

- Professor Department of Ophthalmology, Faculty of Clinical Medicine Mannheim of the University Heidelberg, Germany

K. Schwartz MD

- Bascom Palmer Eye Institute, Miami, USA

Karim F. Damji, MD, FRCSC

- Associate Professor The University of Ottawa Eye Institute and the Ottawa Health Research Institute, Ottawa, Ontario, Canada

Kuldev Singh, MD, MPH

- Associate Professor of Ophthalmology, Director of Glaucoma Service Stanford University, California, USA

L. Jay Katz, MD

- Professor of Ophthalmology Attending Surgeon Glaucoma Service, Co-Director Glaucoma Service, Wills Eye Hospital/Jefferson Medical College, Philadelphia, USA

Leonard A. Levin, MD, PhD

- Associate Professor, Department of Ophthalmology and Visual Sciences, University of Wisconsin Medical School, Madison, USA

Lili Farrokh-Siar, MD

- University Eye Specialists Chicago Center for Vision Research and the Department of Ophthalmology, Northwestern University Chicago, USA

Linda Zangwill, PhD

- Associate Professor, Diagnostic Imaging Laboratory, Hamilton Glaucoma Center Department of Ophthalmology, University of California, San Diego, CA, USA

M. Bruce Shields, MD

- Professor and Chairman, Department of Ophthalmology and Visual Science Yale University School of Medicine, New Haven, CT, USA

Makoto Araie, MD, PhD

- Professor and Chairman, Department of Ophthalmology, University of Tokyo Graduate School of Medicine, Japan

Marcelo T. Nicolela, MD

- Associate Professor, Department of Ophthalmology, Dalhousie University, Halifax, Canada

Michal Schwartz, PhD

- Professor, Department of Neurobiology, The Weizmann Institute of Science, Rehovot, Israel

Michelle Colev, MD

- University Eye Specialists Chicago Center for Vision Research and the Department of Ophthalmology, Northwestern University Chicago, USA

Monica M. Carrillo, MD

- Department of Ophthalmology, Dalhousie University, Halifax, Nova Scotia, Canada

Neeru Gupta, MD, PhD, FRCSC

- Director of Glaucoma Assistant Professor, Department of Ophthalmology and Vision Sciences, Department of Laboratory Medicine & Pathobiology, University of Toronto, St. Michael's Hospital, Toronto, USA

P. T. Khaw, PhD, FRCP, FRCS, FRCOphth, FRCPath, FIBiol, FMedSci

- Professor of Glaucoma and Ocular Healing & Consultant Ophthalmic Surgeon Director, ORB Ocular Repair and Regeneration Biology, Glaucoma, Pathology and Cell Biology, Moorfields Eye Hospital and Institute of Ophthalmology, England

Pamela A. Sample, PhD

- Professor, Visual Function Laboratory, Hamilton Glaucoma Center, University of California at San Diego, USA

Parag A. Gokhale, MD

- Assistant Professor, Director of the Glaucoma Service, Medical College of Georgia, USA

Paul F. Palmberg, MD, PhD

- Professor of Ophthalmology, Bascom Palmer Eye Institute, Miller School of Medicine, University of Miami, USA

Paul T. K. Chew, FRCS(Ed), FRCOphth

- Associated Professor, Head and Consultant, Glaucoma Service, Singapore National Eye Center, National University of Singapore, National University Hospital, Singapore

Philip P. Chen, MD

- Associate Professor, University of Washington Department of Ophthalmology, Seattle, Washington, USA. Chief of Ophthalmology, University of Washington Medical Center, USA

Raymond P. LeBlanc, MD, FRCSC

- Professor and Head, Department of Ophthalmology, Dalhousie University, Halifax, Nova Scotia, Canada

Richard K. Parrish, MD

- Professor Associated Dean for Graduate Medical Education, Bascom Palmer Eye Institute University of Miami, Miami, Florida, USA

Richard P. Mills, MD, MPH

- Clinical Professor, University of Washington, Seattle, Washington, USA

Roger A. Hitchings, MD, FRCS, FRCOp

- Professor of Glaucoma, Glaucoma Department, Moorfields Eye Hospital/ Institute of Ophthalmology, London, England

Robert D. Fechtner, MD

- Professor Director, Glaucoma Division, New Jersey Medical School, UMDNJ, Newark, USA

Robert Feldman MD

- Clinical Associate Professor, Director of Glaucoma, Hermann Eye Center Memorial Hermann Hospital, Houston, Texas, USA

Robert L. Stamper, MD

- Professor of Clinical Ophthalmology, Director Glaucoma Service, Department of Ophthalmology, University of California, San Francisco, USA

Robert Ritch, FACS

- Surgeon Director and Chief of Glaucoma Services at the New York Eye and Ear Infirmary New York City and Professor of Clinical Ophthalmology at the New York City Medical College, Valhalla, New York

Roberto Freire Santiago Malta, MD

- Professor Associated, University of São Paulo, Brazil from the Department of Clinical Ophthalmology, Medicine Faculty, University of São Paulo, Brazil

Roberto G. Carassa, MD

- Glaucoma Service Department of Ophthalmology and Visual Sciences HS Raffaele, University of Milano, Italia

Roberto M. Vessani, MD

- Preceptor of Service of Glaucoma, Department of Ophthalmology, University of São Paulo, Brazil

S. Fabian Lerner, MD

- Director, Glaucoma Section, Postgraduate Department Favaloro University, School of Medicine, Buenos Aires, Argentina

Shan Lin, MD

- Assistant Professor, Department of Ophthalmology, University of California, USA

Stephen M. Drance, MD

- Emeritus Professor, Department of Ophthalmology, University of British Columbia, Vancouver BC, Canada

Steve K. L. Seah, FRCS(Ed), FRCOphth

- Head and Senior Consultant, Glaucoma Service, Singapore National Eye Centre, Singapore

Theodore Krupin, MD

- Clinical Professor, University Eye Specialists Chicago Center for Vision Research and the Department of Ophthalmology, Northwestern University Chicago, USA

Tin Aung, FRCS (Ed), FRCOpth

- Consultant, Singapore National Eye Center National University of Singapore National University Hospital, Singapore

Tony Realini, MD

- Associate Professor, Department of Ophthalmology, University of West Virginia, West Virginia, USA

Troy M. Tanji, MD

- Assistant Clinical Professor of Surgery, Division of Ophthalmology, University of Hawaii John A. Burns School of Medicine, Honolulu, Hawaii

Tsing-Hong Wang, MD, PhD

- Department of Ophthalmology National Taiwan University Hospital Taipei, Taiwan

Vincent Hugo, MD

- Department of Ophthalmology, The New York Eye And Ear Infirmary, New York, USA

Wallace L. M. Alward, MD

- Professor and Vice-Chairman Director, Glaucoma Service University of Iowa College of Medicine Iowa City, Iowa, USA

Yeni H. Yücel, MD, PhD, FRCPC

- Assistant Professor, Department of Ophthalmology and Vision Sciences, Department of Laboratory Medicine & Pathobiology, University of Toronto, St. Michael's Hospital, Toronto, Canada

Preface

For this book, we sought to compile a series of questions that probe the current condition of the conundrum of glaucoma. Many of the answers that have been provided by the invited experts are definitive and based on clinical or laboratory research that has become possible due to the emergence of new technologies and methodologies. Others express opinions that are anecdotal and based on experience or logic. It was our intent that these questions and the elicited responses would not only provide didactic information about glaucoma, but raise new questions. Some of the new questions might be designed to elucidate existing answers. Others might arise from the surprise of learning something inconsistent with previous expectations or understandings. And still others might arise from either practical need or curiosity. An enhanced understanding of glaucoma depends upon the generation of answers to these new questions, as well as informed alterations of the answers to the existing ones provided here.

Remo Susanna Jr. MD

São Paulo, Brazil

Robert N. Weinreb MD

La Jolla, USA

Contents

Question 1

How is glaucoma defined?

Robert N. Weinreb

Felipe A. Medeiros

Glaucoma is a progressive optic neuropathy with characteristic structural changes in the optic nerve head, frequently accompanied by corresponding changes in the visual field. It has diverse etiologies, including those which are idiopathic. Moreover, there are a variety of factors, including the intraocular pressure (IOP), that increase the risk of developing glaucoma. Glaucomatous optic neuropathy can be defined as a final common pathway for a group of conditions which share common biological properties and clinical characteristics.

Biological definition

Glaucomatous optic neuropathy results from specific pathophysiological changes in retinal ganglion cell axons, also known as optic nerve fibers.[1-3] Characteristic morphological changes in the glaucomatous optic nerve are thought to originate at the level of the lamina cribrosa. There is compression and posterior displacement of this lamina and axonal damage. Studies in cats and monkeys with experimentally induced ocular hypertension have demonstrated blockade of both orthograde and retrograde axonal transport at the level of the lamina cribrosa. This results in collections of vesicles and mitochondria with disorganization of microtubules and neurofilaments at the posterior level of the lamina cribrosa. In post-mortem surgery on human eyes with primary open-angle glaucoma, similar ultrastructural changes in optic nerve fibers have been observed, which are consistent with the experimental observations.

Whether glaucomatous optic neuropathy can result from only an intraocular pressure which is sufficiently high is not known. In some cases, impaired microcirculation, altered immunity, excitotoxicity, and other factors, either separately or in combination with intraocular pressure, may also contribute.[1] Regardless of the cause, a cascade of specific events – compression and posterior displacement of the lamina cribrosa, retinal ganglion cell axonal transport disruption and subsequent selective degeneration of optic nerve fibers – leads to glaucomatous optic nerve damage. This cascade is what appears to distinguish glaucomatous neuropathy from other optic neuropathies at the cellular level.

Clinical definition

From a clinical perspective, glaucoma is a progressive optic neuropathy with characteristic structural damage that is frequently accompanied by a specific type of visual field defect. Although the level of IOP is one of the most consistent risk factors for the presence of glaucoma, several population-based studies have documented optic disc and visual field damage characteristic of glaucoma in individuals with statistically normal IOP. Conversely, a large number of people with statistically raised IOP do not develop glaucoma even during lengthy follow-up.

Structural changes

With retinal ganglion cell death and nerve fiber loss in glaucoma, particular structural changes in the appearance of the optic nerve head and retinal nerve fiber layer are observed.[4] Axonal loss results in progressive neuroretinal rim thinning and excavation of the optic nerve head. Although progressive excavation is the characteristic change noted in the glaucomatous optic nerve head, other changes may be suspicious, including vertical elongation of the cup, notching of the neuroretinal rim, presence of asymmetry in the cup-to-disc ratio measurements between the two eyes, splinter hemorrhage, parapapillary atrophy and regional pallor. Progressive retinal nerve fiber layer changes, in a localized and/or diffuse pattern, can be observed concomitantly with changes in the optic nerve head. Occasionally, non-glaucomatous optic neuropathies are diagnosed incorrectly as glaucomatous. Unlike other optic neuropathies, the glaucomatous optic nerve head is excavated and the excavation typically exceeds the extent of pallor.

Functional changes

Glaucoma affects several aspects of the visual function. The best known functional consequence of glaucoma is the progressive deterioration of visual field which usually begins in the midperiphery, often in the superior field, and may progress in a centripetal manner to result in a remaining central or temporal island of vision in advanced cases. These characteristic visual field defects correspond topographically to the retinal nerve fiber layer loss. Although deficits in visual function are usually considered as part of the definition of glaucoma, several studies have demonstrated that glaucomatous changes to the optic disc or retinal nerve fiber layer can often precede the development of visual field defects as assessed by standard automated perimetry.[5-7]

Other functional changes in glaucoma include loss of color sensitivity, especially for short-wavelength (blue) light, as well as loss of spatial resolution, motion detection and temporal contrast sensitivity. Testing for loss of sensitivity of blue light with short-wavelength automated perimetry (SWAP) has been demonstrated to be more sensitive for diagnosing and monitoring glaucomatous visual field loss than standard automated perimetry.[8-11] Frequency doubling technology perimetry also seems to be more sensitive for detecting early changes in visual function in glaucoma.[12,13] Although many of these changes have been observed to occur years before abnormalities in standard perimetry are noted, these tests have not been widely used in clinical practice.

Case definition of glaucoma

There is a lack of consistency on how glaucoma is defined. This is illustrated by a literature review of articles published on open-angle glaucoma (OAG) in 3 major ophthalmic journals. One hundred and eighty two articles were reviewed to identify optic nerve, visual field, and IOP criteria used to define glaucoma. Of the 182 articles, 120 (66%) included a definition of OAG. Among these, approximately 36% used both optic disc and visual field criteria, 13% used optic disc or visual field criteria, 26% used only visual field criteria, 20% used only IOP, and 5% used only optic disc criteria.[14]

The absence of a consensus definition impedes research in glaucoma. It prevents accurate estimation of prevalence estimates and the accumulation of valid clinical evidence on the effectiveness of treatment or risk factors for the disease. The effect of applying different commonly used criteria for diagnosis of open angle glaucoma has been examined.[15] Prevalence figures ranging from 0.1% to 1.2% in the same population were identified. The use of study specific case definitions impairs the interpretation and comparison of research results. Table 1 summarizes definitions for glaucoma used in some major epidemiological studies. As a result of different definitions use for diagnosis, the results from these studies are difficult to compare, hampering meta-analyses and evaluation of risk factors.

The lack of a detailed case definition for glaucoma that can be applied in clinical practice results in considerable uncertainty about the diagnosis of this condition. This can lead to unnecessary lifelong treatment and follow-up for someone being misdiagnosed with this incurable disease, possibly resulting in a significant negative impact on his/her mental or physical (from treatment side effects) health. On the other hand, the lack of knowledge about the clinical features of the disease, including the characteristic signs of glaucomatous damage to the optic nerve, can result in late diagnosis and irreversible loss of visual function.

Table 1. Different criteria used for definition of open angle glaucoma in major epidemiological surveys.*

Baltimore Eye Survey[16]	Optic disc criteria (CDR ≥ 0.8, or asymmetry ≥ 0.3 between both eyes) associated with VF defect not explained by other causes. No IOP criterion.
Barbados Eye Study[17]	Definite glaucoma: At least 2 abnormal VF associated with 2 of 3 of the following criteria: CDR ≥ 0.7, asymmetry ≥ 0.2, rim width ≤ 0.1, notching or disc hemorrhage.
Beaver Dam Eye Study[18]	At least two of the following criteria: VF defect not explained by other causes, CDR ≥ 0.8 or asymmetry in CDR ≥ 0.2, IOP ≥ 22 mmHg, or IOP-lowering treatment.
Blue Mountains Eye Study[19]	Glaucomatous VF defect not explained by other causes, combined with vertical CDR ≥ 0.7 or asymmetry in vertical CDR ≥ 0.3 between both eyes.
Egna-Neumarkt Eye Study[20]	At least 2 of the following criteria: glaucomatous VF defect, IOP ≥ 22mmHg and 1 of the following: CDR ≥ 0.7, CDR asymmetry > 0.2, difference in vertical and horizontal CDR >0.2, or notching, or disc hemorrhage, or excavation reaching disc margin.
Framingham Study[21]	VF defect not explained by other causes, combined with vertical CDR ≥ 0.6 or CDR asymmetry ≥ 0.2.
Los Angeles Latino Eye Study[22]	Glaucomatous VF defects and/or characteristic optic disc damage as assessed by stereophotographs. No IOP criterion.
Rotterdam Study[15]	Definite glaucoma: Glaucomatous VF defect associated with vertical CDR ≥ 0.7, or asymmetry ≥ 0.2 between both eyes, or minimal rim width < 0.1.

* CDR – cup-to-disc ratio; VF – visual field

REFERENCES

1. Weinreb RN, Khaw PT. Primary open-angle glaucoma. Lancet 2004;363:1711-20.

2. Medeiros FA, Weinreb RN. Medical backgrounders: glaucoma. Drugs Today (Barc) 2002;38:563-70.

3. Fechtner RD, Weinreb RN. Mechanisms of optic nerve damage in primary open angle glaucoma. Surv Ophthalmol 1994;39:23-42.

4. Jonas JB, Budde WM, Panda-Jonas S. Ophthalmoscopic evaluation of the optic nerve head. Surv Ophthalmol 1999;43:293-320.

5. Quigley HA, Dunkelberger GR, Green WR. Retinal ganglion cell atrophy correlated with automated perimetry in human eyes with glaucoma. Am J Ophthalmol 1989;107:453-64.

6. Sommer A, Katz J, Quigley HA, et al. Clinically detectable nerve fiber atrophy precedes the onset of glaucomatous field loss. Arch Ophthalmol 1991;109:77-83.

7. Harwerth RS, Carter-Dawson L, Smith EL, 3rd, Barnes G, Holt WF, Crawford ML. Neural losses correlated with visual losses in clinical perimetry. Invest Ophthalmol Vis Sci 2004;45:3152-60.

8. Sample PA, Weinreb RN. Color perimetry for assessment of primary open-angle glaucoma. Invest Ophthalmol Vis Sci 1990;31:1869-75.

9. Sample PA, Taylor JD, Martinez GA, Lusky M, Weinreb RN. Short-wavelength color visual fields in glaucoma suspects at risk. Am J Ophthalmol 1993;115:225-33.

10. Johnson CA, Adams AJ, Casson EJ, Brandt JD. Blue-on-yellow perimetry can predict the development of glaucomatous visual field loss. Arch Ophthalmol 1993;111:645-50.

11. Johnson CA, Adams AJ, Casson EJ, Brandt JD. Progression of early glaucomatous visual field loss as detected by blue-on-yellow and standard white-on-white automated perimetry. Arch Ophthalmol 1993;111:651-6.

12. Landers JA, Goldberg I, Graham SL. Detection of early visual field loss in glaucoma using frequency-doubling perimetry and short-wavelength automated perimetry. Arch Ophthalmol 2003;121:1705-10.

13. Medeiros FA, Sample PA, Weinreb RN. Frequency doubling technology perimetry abnormalities as predictors of glaucomatous visual field loss. Am J Ophthalmol 2004;137:863-71.

14. Bathija R, Gupta N, Zangwill L, Weinreb RN. Changing definition of glaucoma. J Glaucoma 1998;7:165-9.

15. Wolfs RC, Borger PH, Ramrattan RS, et al. Changing views on open-angle glaucoma: definitions and prevalences—The Rotterdam Study. Invest Ophthalmol Vis Sci 2000;41:3309-21.

16. Tielsch JM, Katz J, Singh K, et al. A population-based evaluation of glaucoma screening: the Baltimore Eye Survey. Am J Epidemiol 1991;134:1102-10.

17. Leske MC, Connell AM, Schachat AP, Hyman L. The Barbados Eye Study. Prevalence of open angle glaucoma. Arch Ophthalmol 1994;112:821-9.

18. Klein BE, Klein R, Sponsel WE, et al. Prevalence of glaucoma. The Beaver Dam Eye Study. Ophthalmology 1992;99:1499-504.

19. Mitchell P, Smith W, Attebo K, Healey PR. Prevalence of open-angle glaucoma in Australia. The Blue Mountains Eye Study. Ophthalmology 1996;103:1661-9.

20. Bonomi L, Marchini G, Marraffa M, et al. Prevalence of glaucoma and intraocular pressure distribution in a defined population. The Egna-Neumarkt Study. Ophthalmology 1998;105:209-15.

21. Kahn HA, Milton RC. Alternative definitions of open-angle glaucoma. Effect on prevalence and associations in the Framingham eye study. Arch Ophthalmol 1980;98:2172-7.

22. Varma R, Ying-Lai M, Francis BA, et al. Prevalence of open-angle glaucoma and ocular hypertension in Latinos: the Los Angeles Latino Eye Study. Ophthalmology 2004;111:1439-48.

Question 2

Why do people go blind from glaucoma?

Monica M. Carrillo

Raymond P. LeBlanc

Given the pace of new technological applications in glaucoma management, and the collective information that recent glaucoma trials have provided to make informed decisions on when and how to treat glaucoma, it is important to identify those areas that warrant close attention to prevent blindness from glaucoma. Glaucoma is the leading cause of blindness among adult African-Americans[1] and the second leading cause of blindness worldwide after cataract, with nearly 7.6 million persons throughout the world estimated to be bilaterally blind according to the World Health Organization standard of <20/400.[2] Unlike cataract blindness, glaucoma blindness is irreversible. Bilateral blindness affects less than 10% of those with open angle glaucoma, but 25 to 30% of angle closure glaucoma sufferers.[2,3]

The reason glaucoma causes blindness in so many cases is that most individuals do not notice the visual field loss until significant optic nerve damage has already occurred and some vision is lost. It has been estimated that in industrialized countries, one-half of all patients with glaucoma do not know that they have the disease and are consequently not receiving treatment that may prevent vision loss.[1,3] In the developing world, 90 to 100% of those affected are unaware that they have the disease and, when blind, do not know what has caused their impairment.[2,4] While in the latter communities this could respond to the fact that the costs of standard methods of glaucoma screening are prohibitive and subsequently glaucoma is not included in health care delivery nor is it a public health priority thus almost all cases remain unidentified, there is no justification for the failure to

9

diagnose glaucoma in almost half of those affected in Europe, North America, and Australia.

Population studies have shown that increased intraocular pressure leads to an increase in the incidence[5] and prevalence[6,7] of glaucoma. It is clear from recent glaucoma trials[8-14] that while treatment to lower IOP will minimize the rate of progression of optic nerve damage and subsequently glaucoma-related blindness, IOP alone is not responsible for the disease. The Collaborative Normal Tension Glaucoma Study (CNTGS) group[9], Advanced Glaucoma Intervention Study (AGIS)[8], Collaborative Initial Glaucoma Treatment Study (CIGTS)[11], Ocular Hypertension Treatment Study (OHTS)[12] and Early Manifest Glaucoma Trial (EMGT)[13] are all gold standard prospective, randomized clinical trials that support this concept. Risk factors for glaucoma progression identified in these glaucoma trials are outlined in Table 1. This information can be incorporated into models that calculate the risk of developing glaucomatous visual loss. These models will certainly need constant refinement and improvement as we learn more from ongoing and future trials.

Unfortunately, in some cases, blindness from glaucoma can occur despite therapy. Long-term studies have shown that a significant number of glaucoma patients can experience disease progression despite clinically acceptable IOP reduction.[8,15,16] Currently, IOP is the only component of glaucoma that we can treat, as neuro-protective therapy has not yet been validated as safe and effective. The individual susceptibility of glaucomatous eyes to different IOP levels indicates that establishment of a target IOP and ongoing monitoring of glaucomatous damage are critical in a modern glaucoma practice. Such target pressures should be adjusted if the patient's condition changes.

Additionally, it is essential to identify high-risk individuals who should be treated from lower risk individuals who may be able to be followed without treatment until a defined event suggestive of misclassification occurs.

In nearly all cases, blindness from glaucoma is preventable. This prevention requires the development of efficient, accurate methods for glaucoma screening to detect those patients at greatest risk, further awareness of glaucoma risk factors among the public, and in those diagnosed with glaucoma, adequate therapy, continued monitoring of the optic nerve, retinal nerve fiber layer and perimetric performance and reassessment of target intraocular pressure levels whenever progression becomes evident.

Table 1. Risk Factors Associated with Glaucoma Progression

1. CNTGS[9]
Female gender
Migraine
Raynauds disease
2. OHTS[10]
Older age
Race (African American)
Sex (male)
Vertical cup-disc ratio
Elevated IOP
Higher visual field pattern standard deviation
Thinner central corneal measurements
3. EMGT[13]
Baseline IOP
Pseudoexfoliation
Greater visual field mean deviation
Age
Presence of disc hemorrhages
4. Other studies
Vascular risk factors (nocturnal hypotension, diabetes, previous vein occlusion)
Family history of or genetic mutation predisposing to glaucoma
Presence and severity of damage to involved or fellow eye
Large fluctuation or instability in IOP
Axial myopia

REFERENCES

1. American Academy of Ophthalmology . Preferred practice pattern: primary open-angle glaucoma. San Francisco, Calif, 1996.

2. Quigley H. How common is glaucoma worldwide? International Glaucoma Review, 2002:11-12.

3. Quigley HA. Number of people with glaucoma worldwide. Br J Ophthalmol, 1996; 80:389-93.

4. Robin A. Developing world problems in ophthalmology. Worldwide glaucoma, 2000:12.

5. Sommer A, Tielsch JM, Katz J et al. Relationship between intraocular pressure and primary open angle glaucoma among white and black Americans. The Baltimore Eye Survey. Arch Ophthalmol, 1991;109:1090-5.

6. Leske MC, Connell AM, Wu SY, Hyman LG, Schachat AP. Risk factors for open-angle glaucoma. The Barbados Eye Study. Arch Ophthalmol, 1995;113:918-24.

7. Armaly MF, Krueger DE, Maunder L et al. Biostatistical analysis of the collaborative glaucoma study. I. Summary report of the risk factors for glaucomatous visual-field defects. Arch Ophthalmol, 1980;98:2163-71.

8. The Advanced Glaucoma Intervention Study (AGIS): 7. The relationship between control of intraocular pressure and visual field deterioration.The AGIS Investigators. Am J Ophthalmol, 2000;130:429-40.

9. Drance S, Anderson DR, Schulzer M. Risk factors for progression of visual field abnormalities in normal-tension glaucoma. Am J Ophthalmol, 2001;131:699-708.

10. Gordon MO, Beiser JA, Brandt JD et al. The Ocular Hypertension Treatment Study: baseline factors that predict the onset of primary open-angle glaucoma. Arch Ophthalmol, 2002;120:714-20; discussion 829-30.

11. Janz NK, Wren PA, Lichter PR et al. The Collaborative Initial Glaucoma Treatment Study: interim quality of life findings after initial medical or surgical treatment of glaucoma. Ophthalmology, 2001;108:1954-65.

12. Kass MA, Heuer DK, Higginbotham EJ et al. The Ocular Hypertension Treatment Study: a randomized trial determines that topical ocular hypotensive medication delays or prevents the onset of primary open-angle glaucoma. Arch Ophthalmol, 2002;120:701-13; discussion 829-30.

13. Leske MC, Heijl A, Hussein M, Bengtsson B, Hyman L, Komaroff E. Factors for glaucoma progression and the effect of treatment: the early manifest glaucoma trial. Arch Ophthalmol, 2003;121:48-56.

14. Lichter PR, Musch DC, Gillespie BW et al. Interim clinical outcomes in the Collaborative Initial Glaucoma Treatment Study comparing initial treatment randomized to medications or surgery. Ophthalmology, 2001;108:1943-53.

15. Martinez-Bello C, Chauhan BC, Nicolela MT, McCormick TA, LeBlanc RP. Intraocular pressure and progression of glaucomatous visual field loss. Am J Ophthalmol, 2000; 129:302-8.

16. The effectiveness of intraocular pressure reduction in the treatment of normal-tension glaucoma. Collaborative Normal-Tension Glaucoma Study Group. Am J Ophthalmol, 1998;126:498-505.

Question 3

How often do patients with glaucoma become blind?

Douglas H. Johnson

Glaucoma is the leading cause of irreversible blindness in the world, and the second leading cause of blindness in the world[1]. This data comes from surveys of people who are blind from a variety of causes, and indicates that glaucoma ranks with cataract and trachoma in significance. But what about the flip side to this question: in patients with known glaucoma, how often does it lead to blindness?

How often do patients with glaucoma become blind?

Single screening examinations: Population screening surveys to determine the prevalence of eye disease indicate that about 50% of people with glaucoma are unaware they have the condition. In these screenings, about 4% of white persons and 8% of black persons with glaucoma are blind.[2] This is consistent with the finding that 5% of people with newly diagnosed glaucoma were blind at the time of diagnosis in a long-term study of glaucoma.[3]

Blindness from glaucoma: screening studies

	n	% blind OU from GL* (white pt; visual acuity only)
Baltimore[4]	2913	4.4%
Beaver Dam[1]	4926	2.5%
Ireland[5]	2186	6.2%
Rotterdam[6]	3062	3.0%
Olmsted County[3] (20 yr long-term Rx)	290	5.0%

The definition of blindness is important. Most screening surveys use the World Health Organization definition, which includes only visual acuity and not visual field loss. In the United States, visual field loss is also included, which results in higher rates of blindness.[3]

Long-term follow-up: Screening surveys provide information at only one point in time in a chronic disease process. If patients are followed long-term, the probability of blindness from glaucoma increases. In a longitudinal study of patients living in Olmsted County, Minnesota, patients with disc or field damage at the time of diagnosis had a 54% probability of becoming legally blind in at least one eye, and 22% probability of becoming blind in both eyes after 20 years.[3] In eyes without disc or field damage at the time of diagnosis the risk was lower but not inconsequential: 14% probability of going blind in at least one eye, and 4% risk in becoming blind in both eyes after 20 years. About one-half of the patients in each of these groups were blind from loss of visual acuity, and the other half from field loss alone, with preservation of central acuity.

Early detection can help lower the progression to blindness. A recent study of patients diagnosed with glaucoma by computerized visual field testing (abnormal statistical outcome of the sensitive pattern standard deviation and the Glaucoma Hemifield test on the Humphrey perimeter) found the probability of blindness after 15 years in one eye to be 14.6% and both eyes 6.4%[7]. These patients were in a University practice under the care of glaucoma specialists, differing from the community based population cared for by general ophthalmologists reported in Olmsted County.[3] For comparison, at 15 years, the Olmsted rates were 20% probability in one eye and 6% in both eyes overall, with higher rates among eyes with significant damage at the time of diagnosis of glaucoma.[3]

Why do some people go blind from glaucoma?

Progression rates appear to be dependent upon intraocular pressure levels, as described in the AGIS study.[8] Progression rates are not necessarily linear, as evidenced by the finding that up to 40% of axons can be lost before disc or field changes are evident.[9] *Patients becoming blind have faster rates of progression than those who do not, and assessing rates of field progression by using simple group averages loses the ability to track fast progressors,* especially if the study is short-term and does not follow patients to blindness.[10,11]

Blindness in patients with known glaucoma may occur because of patient non-compliance, or treatment failures. Treatment failures can result: 1) when therapy is not aggressive enough in lowering intraocular pressure, 2) progression of disease is not recognized or responded to soon enough, or 3) in some cases disease can progress despite aggressive treatment efforts.

Achieving a low enough intraocular pressure to prevent further damage remains the mainstay of treatment. Most studies use a goal of lowering IOP about 20% after damage is detected. Another approach would be to determine a patient's target IOP based upon the amount of damage, regardless of the initial IOP at the time of diagnosis. *Most important in treatment is to reassess each patient in light of ongoing glaucomatous damage, with additional lowering of the IOP goal required each time progression is found.* Although medications to protect or strengthen the optic nerve hold promise for the future, current therapy requires adequate lowering of intraocular pressure.

REFERENCES

1. Quigley HA. The number of people with glaucoma worldwide. Br J Ophthalmol, 1996; 80:389-393.

2. Sommer A, Tielsch JM, Katz J, et al: Racial differences in the cause-specific prevalence of blindness in east Baltimore. N Engl J Med, 1991;325:1412-11417.

3. Hattenhauer MG, Johnson DH, Ing HH, Herman DC, Hodge DO: The probability of blindness from open angle glaucoma. Ophthalmology, 105:2099-2104, 1998

4. Sommer A, Tielsch JM, Katz J, Royall RM, Quigley HA, et al. Racial differences in the cause-specific prevalence of blindness in east Baltimore N Engl J Med, 1991; 325:1412-1417.

5. Coffey M, Reidy A, Wormald R, Xian WX, Wright L, Courtney P. Prevalence of glaucoma in the west of Ireland. Br J Ophthalmol, 1993;77:17-21.

6. Dielemans I, Vingerling JR, Wolfs RC, Hofman A, Grobbee DE, deJong PT. The prevalence of primary open-angle glaucoma in a population-based study in the Netherlands. Ophthalmology, 1994;101:1851-1855.

7. Chen PP. Blindness in patients with treated open angle glaucoma. Ophthalmology, 2003; 110:726-733.

8. Vanveldhuisen PC, Ederer F, Gaasterland DE et al: AGIS 7: The relationship between control of intraocular pressure and visual field deterioration. Am J Ophthalmol, 2001; 130:429-440.

9. Quigley HA, Addicks KM, Green WR. Optic nerve damage in human glaucoma III. Quantitative correlation of nerve fiber loss and visual field defect. Arch Ophthalmol, 1982;100:135- 146.

10. Oliver JE, Hattenhauer MG, Herman D, Hodge DO, Kennedy R, Fang-Yen M, Johnson DH. Blindness and glaucoma: a comparison of patients progressing to blindness from glaucoma with patients maintaining vision. Am J Ophthalmol, 133:764-772, 2002.

11. Quigley HA, Tielsch JM, Katz J, Sommer A. Rate of progression in open-angle glaucoma estimated from cross-sectional prevalence of visual field damage. Am J Ophthalmol, 1996;122:355-363.

Question 4

What causes optic nerve damage in glaucoma?

Douglas R. Anderson

Glaucomatous cupping is an optic neuropathy in which the level of intraocular pressure (IOP) affects the course of the disease. The prevalence of glaucoma is progressively greater when the IOP is higher. Even in cases of glaucomatous damage that occurs while the IOP is in the statistically normal range, the progression of damage is reduced if the IOP is made lower[1,2,3].

There is considerably variability in the amount of damage, if any, produced by any particular level of IOP. Age, family history, and other clinical features help predict whether a person has, or will develop, glaucoma[4,5,6]. Individual traits interact with intraocular pressure in some manner to make damage more likely and more severe with an elevation of the intraocular pressure, and to permit the process of glaucomatous damage to be slowed or halted by lowering the IOP.

The complete pathogenic process must consist of several contributing physiologic or pathophysiologic components. In addition to damaging the axons, the pathogenic process causes collapse of the lamina cribrosa to produce cupping - - a unique feature of optic atrophy due to glaucoma, rarely seen in non-glaucomatous optic atrophies.

Some features of the process are genetic. Some genes affect the level of intraocular pressure, but likely other genes affect the process, such as those that govern blood flow physiology or a tendency for cardiovascular disease, that affect rates of cellular apoptosis, that affect connective tissue composition, that affect the molecular biology of astroglia and neurons, and so on. Therefore, patients with "normal tension glaucoma" often have a family history of glaucoma, and that population groups with different genetic

17

heritage vary in the prevalence of chronic glaucomatous optic nerve damage, with or without an abnormal IOP.

Age brings not only an increasing IOP in some people, but seemingly a greater tendency for development of cupping and field loss from an elevated IOP (or with a normal IOP). Perhaps neurons and support structures are weaker with age. Perhaps vascular diseases result with age from interplay of genetic predisposition plus life style (diet, exercise, etc).

Females are more often found to have normal tension glaucoma[4], but in the ocular hypertension treatment study[5] and in the early manifest glaucoma treatment study[6], there was no female preponderance. Vasospasm reflects abnormal vascular regulation (dysregulation, or abnormal autoregulation), and inability to adjust blood flow appropriately is another physiologic trait that may lead to susceptibility to damage when IOP challenges the circulation[7,8].

Poor perfusion may also result from vascular occlusive disease, and there is some evidence that glaucomatous damage from this type of vascular disease is less affected by the IOP level than when ischemia is related to abnormal vascular regulation[9,10].

By some combination of various factors, an episode of ischemia may occur, less extensive and perhaps transient (several hours, rather than permanent as occurs in acute anterior ischemic optic neuropathy). Ischemia produces an environment with various free radicals and highly reactive ions that may damage both the axons and the connective tissue of the lamina cribrosa, maybe during the reperfusion phase[7,8]. Added to this, astroglia may produce damaging levels of nitric oxide[11] when subjected to pressure. If axon membranes are damaged and made permeable, calcium enters the cytoplasm and activates calcium-dependent proteases that can destroy the axon.

Milder ischemia may not destroy the axon where it passes through the optic nerve head, but simply reduce the production of ATP. This may impair conduction of an action potential (perhaps producing reversible scotomas in the visual field), but also may interfere with the transport of growth factors to the ganglion cell. If the cell is deprived of growth factors for a critical period of time, apoptosis is triggered and the ganglion cell will destroy itself[12]. As the cells break apart, glutamate is among the substances released, and could be toxic to adjacent ganglion cells, compounding the damage. While evidence for these various molecular and tissue events have been found, the relative importance of each is unknown, nor is it certain that the proportionate contributions of these mechanisms is the same in each individual.

There is still much to learn about the details of how the optic nerve is damaged in glaucoma. When the details are understood more fully, the hope is that traits other than simply the level of IOP will help identify who is at risk of glaucomatous damage, and it can be hoped that therapy can be developed to eliminate the factors that make the optic nerve susceptible to glaucomatous damage or interrupt the cascade of events involved in producing glaucomatous optic atrophy, with or without an elevated intraocular pressure.

REFERENCES

1. Anderson DR, Drance SM, and Schulzer M, writing committee for Collaborative Normal-tension Glaucoma Study Group. Comparison of glaucomatous progression between untreated patients with normal-tension glaucoma and patients with therapeutically reduced intraocular pressures. Amer Jour Ophthalmol, 1998;126:487-497.

2. Anderson DR, Drance SM, and Schulzer M, writing committee for Collaborative Normal-tension Glaucoma Study Group. The effectiveness of intraocular pressure reduction in the treatment of normal-tension glaucoma. Amer Jour Ophthalmol, 1998; 126:498-505.

3. Leske MD, Heijl A, Hussein M, Bengtsson B, Hyman L, and Komaroff E. Factors for glaucoma progression and the effect of treatment. The early manifest glaucoma trial. Arch Ophthalmol, 2003;121:48-56.

4. Anderson DR, Drance SM, and Schulzer, M as writing committee for the Collaborative Normal-Tension Glaucoma Study Group. Risk factors for progression of visual field abnormalities in normal tension glaucoma. American Journal of Ophthalmology, 2001; 131:699-708.

5. Gordon MO, Beiser JA, Brandt JD, Heuer DK, Higginbotham EJ, Johnson CA, Keltner JL, Miller JP, Parrish RK II, et al., for the Ocular Hypertension Treatment Study Group: The Ocular Hypertension Study: Baseline factors that predict the onset of primary open-angle glaucoma. Arch Ophthalmol, 2002;120:714-720.

6. Leske MC, Heijl A, Hussein M, Bengtsson B, Hyman L, Kamaroff E. Factors for glaucoma progression and the effect of treatment. The early manifest glaucoma trial. Arch Ophthalmol, 2003;121:48-56.

7. Flammer J, Pache M, Resink T. Vasospasm, its role in the pathogenesis of diseases with particular reference to the eye. Progress in Retinal and Eye Research, 2001; 20:319-349.

8. Flammer J, Orgul S, Costa VP, Orzalesi N, Krieglstein GK, Serra LM, Renard J-P., and Stefánsson E. The impact of ocular blood flow in glaucoma. Progress in Retinal and Eye Research, 2002;21:359-393.

9. Schulzer M, Drance SM, Carter CJ, Brooks DE, Lau W. Biostatistical evidence for two distinct populations with chronic open angle glaucoma. Br J Ophthalmol, 1990; 74:196-200.

10. Anderson DR, Drance SM, Schulzer M. Factors that predict the benefit of lowering intra-ocular pressure in normal tension glaucoma. Am Jour Ophthalmol, 2003 (in press).

11. Liu B. Neufeld AH. Nitric oxide synthase-2 in human optic nerve head astrocytes induced by elevated pressure in vitro. Arch Ophthal, 2001;119(2):240-5.

12. Kerrigan LA, Zack DJ, Quigley HA, Smith SD, Pease ME. TUNEL-positive ganglion cells in human primary open angle glaucoma. Arch Ophthalmol, 1997;115:1031-5.

Question 5

Selective cell death in glaucoma: does it really exist?

Catherine Boden

Pamela A. Sample

Preferential loss of one retinal ganglion cell (RGC) subtype in early glaucoma – the selective cell death theory – remains controversial.[1,2] Of the more than 20 morphologically and physiologically distinct subtypes of RGCs, 3 are particularly relevant to the continuing debate about the selective cell death theory. These 3 RGC subtypes are known to project to the visual cortex via a relay station called the lateral geniculate nucleus (LGN) (Figure 1).[3] Axons from the small bistratified, magnocellular (M) and parvocellular (P) cells connect to koniocellular, magnocellular and parvocellular layers of the LGN respectively. M and P pathways are not only anatomically and physiologically distinct but also functionally segregated. The M pathway is most sensitive to motion, flicker and high-temporal/low-spatial frequencies, while the P pathway is most sensitive to red-green colour and low-temporal/high-spatial frequencies. Input from the small bistratified RGCs to the koniocellular layers of the LGN is currently believed to carry information about blue-yellow colour but less is known about the K pathway. Although there is some intermixing of input from the subcortical M, P and K pathways at the cortex, the input remains largely separate in visual cortex. The M pathway projects predominantly to the dorsal cortical pathway (motion perception), while the P and K pathways project mostly to the ventral cortical pathway (object perception). This simplified view of the visual system will guide us in understanding the debate about the selective cell death theory.

Some histologic studies have suggested selective loss of larger diameter RGC axons in early glaucoma.[4] Morphologically, M cells tend to have larger axons than the other cell types. Therefore it was postulated that neurons of the M pathway are lost preferentially in glaucoma. Since that time, a debate stemming from conflicting findings and alternative interpretations of the histologic results (Table 1) has been ongoing. Alternative theories of RGC death in glaucoma and predictions based on these theories are described in Table 2.

Newer perimetric tests have been designed to target specific RGC subtypes.[5] These visual-function specific tests are thought to measure the integrity of M-, P- or K-pathways depending upon the test (Figure 1). Standard automated perimetry (SAP) is "non-selective" in that all RGC subtypes can respond to the white flash. If there is selective dropout of M

Table 1. Alternative explanations for evidence supporting selective cell death in glaucoma.

Evidence Supporting Selective Cell Death Theory	Alternative Explanation for the Finding
Histological results from an experimental monkey model of glaucoma – Large diameter retinal ganglion cell axons are more vulnerable to glaucoma.	Size of ganglion cell bodies and axons depends on eccentricity. The small-bistratified cells/axons are larger than those of P-cells. Therefore, the assumption that large axons must be M cells or magnocellular cells may not always be valid.
Histological results from autopsy of human eyes – Relatively greater loss of cells with large axons.	See above. Postmortem shrinkage of axons and dendritic trees alone could account for the histopathological finding without recourse to a selective cell death hypothesis.[12]
Psychophysical results – Visual field defects can be detected earlier with motion tasks. Motion tests are thought to selectively test the M pathway.	Earlier detection of visual field defects by test targeting the M pathway can be explained by reduced redundancy. Psychophysical findings comparing loss of various subtypes in some eyes do not support selective cell loss. There is evidence that both M and P pathways can be involved in motion processing. An early motion deficit could theoretically result from damage to both M and P pathways.

cells in early glaucoma, visual-function specific tests that isolate M pathway function [Frequency Doubling Technology (FDT), motion tests] should show earlier defects than tests that target P or K pathways [high-pass resolution perimetry (HPRP) and SWAP respectively]. Alternatively, visual function specific tests may detect loss earlier than SAP because of reduced redundancy. Only a small proportion of RGCs are sensitive to the stimulus, and the remaining RGCs cannot detect it until brightness or contrast are much higher, unlike SAP where all RGCs can detect the stimulus.

Identification of visual field abnormality by FDT, SWAP and motion-automated perimetry in the same glaucoma patients shows that some patients have defects on SWAP first, others on FDT and still others on motion-automated perimetry.[6] The selective cell death theory is further weakened by two studies comparing field abnormality by a P pathway test (HPRP) with FDT in glaucoma patients, glaucoma suspects and ocular hypertensives.[7,8] There was no difference in the ability of HPRP and FDT to detect visual field abnormality, suggesting P and M pathway loss is similar. Moreover, the psychophysical characteristics of early visual loss do not support the hypothesis that the M pathway is selectively damaged in early glaucoma.[9] Psychophysical results, therefore, suggest the visual pathway affected earliest by glaucoma may depend on the individual.

Experimental glaucoma indicates similar dropout of P and M cells, loss of cells in the parvocellular and magnocellular layers of the LGN and decreased metabolic activity in areas of the visual cortex to which both the M and P pathways project.[10,11] Thus, these recent psychophysical studies in conjunction with histologic studies in experimental glaucoma, more strongly support the "Individual Differences in Selective Cell Death" or "Uniform Cell Death" theories (Table 2). Clinically, we know that visual function specific tests are more sensitive to glaucomatous visual loss than SAP. Field defects, however, may be evident on one test earlier than the others depending upon the patient.[6]

Table 2. Theories of retinal ganglion cell damage by glaucoma. Histological and psychophysical predictions derived from each theory are described, as are example of the clinical implications.

Theory	Description	Prediction	Clinical Implications
Selective Cell Death	Neurons of the M pathway are, for example, lost preferentially in early glaucoma.	*Histological:** Greater loss of RGCs with large cell bodies and axons; greater cell loss in magnocellular layers of the LGN. *Psychophysical:* Visual field defects on motion perimetry and FDT should be detected earlier than for SAP, SWAP or HPRP for all glaucoma patients.	Tailoring perimetric tests to target the M pathway should improve early diagnosis.
Individual Differences in Selective Cell Death	Neurons of a single pathway are selectively affected earlier but individuals differ on whether M, P or K pathway is at earliest risk.	*Histological: * Greater loss of RGCs and optic nerve fibers from a single pathway; greater cell loss in associated layers of the LGN. *Psychophysical:* Visual field defects on visual function specific tests targeting the appropriate pathway should be detected earlier than for SAP or the other visual function specific tests.	Mutliple visual function specific tests may be needed initially to identify early visual field damage.
Uniform Cell Death	Neurons of all M, K and P pathways are equally at risk in early glaucoma.	*Histological: * Uniform loss of RGCs; uniform cell loss in all layers of the LGN. *Psychophysical:* Visual field defects on all visual function specific tests should be detected at the same time and earlier than SAP due to reduced redundancy.	All visual function specific perimetric tests should be equally effective for early detection for all patients.

* Assumes that cell loss occurs at the same rate (once begun) for all RGC subtypes over the course of the disease.

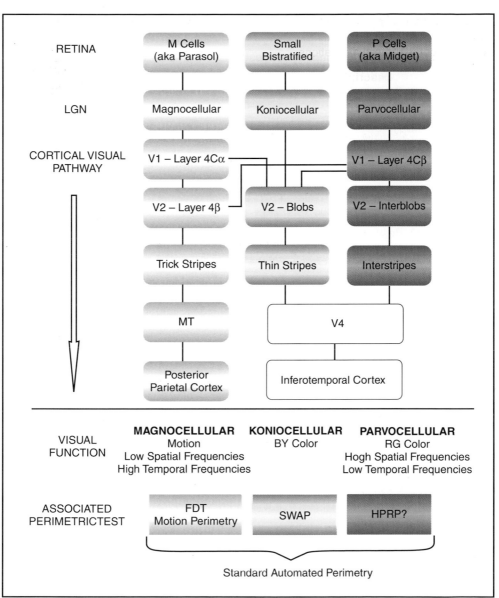

Figure 1. A simple schematic of the parallel visual pathways from the retinal to the cortex. Note that segregation of the M, P and K pathways is largely maintained in the cortex, although in fact there is more intermixing of signals in visual cortices. Visual functions and perimetric tests associated with each pathway are described in the lower third of the schematic. LGN = lateral geniculate nucleus, V1 = visual area 1, V2 = visual area 2, V4 = visual area 4, MT = medial temporal area, FDT = Frequency Doubling Technology Perimetry, SWAP = short-wavelength automated perimetry, HPRP = high pass resolution perimetry.

REFERENCES

1. Hitchings RA. Selective ganglion cell death in glaucoma. British Journal of Ophthalmology, 2000;84(7):678-9.

2. Johnson C. Selective versus non-selective losses in glaucoma. Journal of Glaucoma, 1994;3:S32-S44.

3. Spillman L, Werner JS. Visual Perception. The Neurophysiological Foundations. San Diego: Academic Press Inc, 1990.

4. Quigley HA, Sanchez RM, Dunkelberger GR, et al. Chronic glaucoma selectively damages large optic nerve fibers. Invest Ophthalmol Vis Sci, 1987;28(6):913-20.

5. Sample PA, Bosworth CF, Weinreb RN. The loss of visual function in glaucoma. Seminars in Ophthalmology, 2000;15:182-93.

6. Sample PA, Bosworth CF, Blumenthal EZ, et al. Visual function-specific perimetry for indirect comparison of different ganglion cell populations in glaucoma. Investigative Ophthalmology & Visual Science, 2000;41:1783-9.

7. Martin L, Wanger P, Vancea L, Gothlin B. Concordance of high-pass resolution perimetry and frequency-doubling technology perimetry results in glaucoma: No support for selective ganglion cell damage. Journal of Glaucoma, 2003;12(1):40-4.

8. Kalaboukhova L, Lindblom B. Frequency doubling technology and high-pass resolution perimetry in glaucoma and ocular hypertension. Acta Ophthalmologica Scandinavica, 2003;81(3):247-52.

9. Ansari EA, Morgan JE, Snowden RJ. Psychophysical characterisation of early functional loss in glaucoma and ocular hypertension. British Journal of Ophthalmology, 2002;86(10):1131-5.

10. Crawford MLJ, Harwerth RS, Smith EL, et al. Glaucoma in primates: Cytochrome oxidase reactivity in parvo- and magnocellular pathways. Investigative Ophthalmology & Visual Science, 2000;41(7):1791-802.

11. Yucel YH, Zhang QA, Weinreb RN, et al. Effects of retinal ganglion cell loss on magno-, parvo-, koniocellular pathways in the lateral geniculate nucleus and visual cortex in glaucoma. Progress in Retinal and Eye Research, 2003;22(4):465-81.

12. Morgan JE, Uchida H, Caprioli J. Retinal ganglion cell death in experimental glaucoma. British Journal of Ophthalmology, 2000;84(3):303-10.

Question 6

Is glaucoma only an eye disease?

Stephen M. Drance

The more interesting debate pertains to chronic open angle glaucoma, which was considered in the 1950-60s by most of us as a disease of elevated eye pressure but Dule-Elder and his school felt that the glaucomatous eye was "a sick eye in a sick body."

Numerous population based studies since then have agreed that while the IOP levels in open angle glaucoma patients were higher than among non glaucomatous individuals from 25% to 70% of glaucomatous eyes showed no IOP elevations and the term LTG[1,2] and latterly the term NTG described them. It became clearer that chronic open angle glaucoma was a multifactorial disease. IOP was confirmed as a causative, dose related, major risk factor but was not the only one. The course of glaucoma in patients with elevated pressures was found to be favourably influenced by IOP reduction[3]. Even in NTG the 30% lowering of the statistically normal pressures had a beneficial effect on the disease[4,5] yet up to 20% of patients continued to progress in spite of a marked lowering of their pressures while close to 50% of the untreated patients did not progress[6]. This seems to indicate that some patients have a non, or less, pressure dependent disease than others.

The Baltimore studies[2] demonstrated that glaucoma occurs at all levels of IOP but the higher the pressure the greater its influence while the lower the pressure the more likely the non pressure dependent factors are operative. The course of untreated NTG was shown to be accelerated by gender, race, the presence of a history of migraine and the presence of baseline disc haemorrhages[7].

Glaucoma patients with a wide range of IOP fell into two clusters, one with predominantly vasospastic phenomena was related to IOP produced damage, while the other cluster showed predominantly the presence of

27

laboratory risk factors of vascular disease and damage was not, or much less, related to their highest IOP[8]. Electrocardiographic evidence of ischemic heart disease, which was not used in the clustering of these patients, occurred almost entirely in the cluster with little or no vasospasm. This study suggested a pressure dependent glaucoma and pressure independent (or less dependent) glaucoma. The cases of NTG and POAG were equally distributed in both these clusters.

The clinically varying disc appearances of glaucoma patients also relate to systemic factors[9] including, gender, migraine, vasospasm, systemic hypertension and ischaemic vascular disease. This also suggests that variations in the clinical appearances, their mode of progression, the varying severity of the untreated course of the disease may depend on the presence or absence of the many known, and yet unknown, risk factors in what is clinically recognised as glaucoma. It is hardly surprising that there are conflicting findings in studied groups of glaucoma patients as they will certainly vary, by chance alone, in the presence or absence of certain risk factors. The list of reported vascular abnormalities in glaucoma patients is lengthy and includes ocular and carotid arteriosclerosis, vascular hypertension and hypotension, postural and nocturnal hypotension, vasospasm, endothelin levels, VEGF and vWf levels, endothelial dysfunctions, silent myocardial ischemia, autonomic nervous dysfunction, immune system anomalies, hypothyroidism, diabetes, smoking, sleep disturbances, ischemic brain lesions on MRI, the presence of neurodegenerative diseases such as Alzheimers and Parkinsonism as well as psychiatric disorders. The understanding of the importance of these, and yet to be discovered risk factors, will become clearer in the not too distant future but the notion of the "sick eye in the sick body" should already have implications for the understanding and management of the chronic open angle glaucomas.

REFERENCES

1. Shiose Y, Kitazawa Y, Tsukahara S. et al. Epidemiology of Glaucoma in Japan. Jpn J Ophthalmol, 35,133-155;1991.

2. Tielsch JM, Katz J, Simgh K et al A population based evaluation of glauxoma screening: the Baltimore Eye Survey. Am J Epidemiol, 134,1702-1710;1991.

3. Heijl A, Leske MC, Bengtsson B et al Reduction of intraocular pressure amd glaucoma progression; results from the Early Manifest Glaucoma Trial. Arch Ophthalmol, 120,1268-1279;2002.

4. Collaborative NTG Study Group. Comparison of glaucomatous progression between untreated patients with NTG and patients with therapeutically reduced IOP. Am J Ophthalmol 1998;126: 487-497. [Published erratum appears in Am J Ophthalmol, 1999 Jan;127(1):120].

5. Collaborative NTG Study Group. The effectiveness of IOP reduction in the treatment of NTG. Am J Ophthalmol, 1998;126: 498-505.

6. Collaborative NTG Study Group. Natural History of Normal Tension Glaucoma. Ophthalmology, 108,247-253;2001.

7. Collaborative Normal-Tension Glaucoma Study Group. Risk factors for progression of visual field abnormalities in normal tension glaucoma. Am J Ophthalmol, 2001; 131:699-708.

8. Schulzer M, Drance SM, Carter CJ, Brooks DE, Lau W. Biostatistical evidence for two distinct populations with chronic open angle glaucoma. Br J Ophthalmol, 1990; 74:196-200.

9. Broadway DC, Nicolela MT, Drance SM. Disc appearance in primary open angle glaucoma. Surv Ophthalmol, 1999; 43: S223-S243.

Question 7

Is glaucoma an eye disease only?

Neeru Gupta

Yeni H. Yücel

Glaucoma is considered to be an eye disease with the death of retinal ganglion cells (RGCs) as the major pathology. This leads to progressive loss of vision and is often associated with elevated intraocular pressure (IOP). However, there is evidence that suggests that RGC death is followed by changes within the brain. If we examine carefully a RGC, most of its axon is intracranial in location. The RGC cell body is located in the inner retina, while the axon conveying visual information to the brain has prechiasmal, chiasmal and postchiasmal components. Thus, RGCs are actually not confined to the eye, and the pathological processes contributing to RGC degeneration are likely to be occurring at these intracranial axon components. The first major connecting center located deep within the brain is the lateral geniculate nucleus (LGN). Experimental evidence shows significant degeneration of LGN neurons in glaucoma. The spread of disease from sick neurons to healthy neurons through synaptic connections called trans-synaptic degeneration, as seen in Alzheimer's disease,[1] and may also contribute to progressive damage in glaucoma. Thus, glaucoma might be considered a degenerative disease of the visual system that begins with RGC death.

Within the LGN, the three major visual pathways are exquisitely organized into 6 layers from ventral to dorsal. Magnocellular neurons (sensitive to motion) are found in layers 1 and 2, parvocellular neurons (sensitive to red/green colored stimulus) are located in layers 3 to 6, and koniocellular neurons (sensitive to blue-yellow stimulus) are sandwiched between and within these principle layers.

In the experimental primate glaucoma model, intraocular pressure (IOP) raised in one eye can create varying degrees of optic nerve damage.

Pathological examination of the LGN reveals marked neural degenerative changes including shrinkage and loss of neurons. [2-5] Quantitative assessment using three-dimensional techniques shows significant neuron degeneration in the LGN in magnocellular and parvocellular layers.[2-4] Furthermore, marked reduction of koniocellular blue-yellow neurons is observed.[5] Thus, optic nerve damage can cause degenerative changes in magno-, parvo-, and koniocellular pathways of the LGN.

The neurons of these major vision pathways project to the visual cortex, where further visual information processing occurs. In glaucoma, using cytochrome oxidase, an activity marker, metabolic changes are observed in the visual cortex with alternating light and dark bands, where light bands correspond to ocular dominance columns of low metabolic activity driven by the glaucomatous eye.[5-7] Furthermore, neurochemical alterations are observed in the visual cortex.[8] These data implicate the retina, optic nerve, LGN and the visual cortex in the pathobiology of glaucoma.[9] As optic nerve damage increases, cell death in magnocellular and parvocellular LGN layers also increases. [5] There is a linear relationship between optic nerve fiber loss and neuron shrinkage in both magnocellular and parvocellular pathways in the LGN.[4] These shrunken, surviving LGN neurons may be dysfunctional and represent a window of opportunity to target therapeutically.

Implications [10]

There is compelling experimental evidence to suggest that as RGC death increases in the eye, increasing degenerative changes also increase within the central visual system at various levels. Recent findings suggest that similar processes occur in human central visual system in glaucoma.[11] The best way to stop disease progression may be to target the RGCs using our current therapies as early as possible.

Understanding the pathological spread of glaucomatous injury from RGCs to major vision stations in the brain may help to explain structural and functional changes in disease progression. The LGN provides essential growth factors and nutrient supplies to the retinal ganglion cells. With advancing optic nerve damage, the loss of neurons in the LGN may further weaken an already susceptible population of RGCs due to growth factor deprivation. In advanced cases, treatments aimed solely at the eye may not be sufficient to retard disease progression. Further studies are needed to understand the mechanisms underlying RGC and target neuron degeneration in glaucoma. As we look for new therapeutic strategies to prevent disease progression, in addition to targeting the RGCs, we might also consider targeting neurons in the brain.

Future studies with a multidisciplinary approach to explore alterations at multiple brain stations in glaucoma, including modern functional neuro-physiological approaches,[12] imaging methodologies[13] and neuropathology, may help us to understand glaucoma as a disease of the visual system, not confined to the eye.

REFERENCES

1. J.H. Su, G. Deng, C.W. Cotman. Transneuronal degeneration in the spread of Alzheimer's disease pathology: immunohistochemical evidence for the transmission of tau hyperphosphorylation. Neurobiol Dis, 4: 365-375,1997.

2. Y.H. Yücel, Q. Zhang, N. Gupta, P.L. Kaufman, and R.N. Weinreb. Loss of neurons in magno and parvocellular layers of the lateral geniculate nucleus in glaucoma. Archives of Ophthalmology, 118: 378-384, 2000.

3. A. J. Weber, H.Chen, W. C. Hubbard, P. L Kaufman. Experimental glaucoma and cell size, density, and number in the primate lateral geniculate nucleus. Investigative Ophthalmology and Visual Science, 41: 1370-1379, 2000.

4. Y.H. Yücel, Q. Zhang, R.N. Weinreb, P.L. Kaufman and N. Gupta. Atrophy of relay neurons in magno-and parvocellular layers of the lateral geniculate nucleus in glaucoma. Investigative Ophthalmology and Visual Science, 42: 3216-3222, 2001.

5. Y.H. Yücel, Q. Zhang, R.N. Weinreb, P.L. Kaufman and N. Gupta. Effects of retinal ganglion cell loss on magno-, parvo-, koniocellular pathways in the lateral geniculate nucleus and visual cortex in glaucoma. Progress in Retinal and Eye Research, 22: 465-481, 2003.

6. Vickers JC, Hof PR, Schumer RA, Wang RF, Podos SM, and Morrison JH. Magnocellular and parvocellular visual pathways are both affected in a macaque monkey model of glaucoma. Aust N Z J Ophthalmol, 25:239-243,1997.

7. M.L. Crawford, R.S. Harwerth, E.L. Smith 3rd, F. Shen and L. Carter-Dawson. Glaucoma in primates: cytochrome oxidase reactivity in parvo- and magnocellular pathways. Investigative Ophthalmology and Visual Science, 41: 1791-1802, 2000.

8. D.Y. Lam, P.L. Kaufman, B.T. Gabelt, E.C. To, J.A. Matsubara. Neurochemical correlates of cortical plasticity after unilateral elevated intraocular pressure in a primate model of glaucoma. Investigative Ophthalmology and Visual Science, 44: 2573-2581, 2003.

9. N. Gupta and Y.H. Yücel. Brain changes in glaucoma. European Journal of Ophthalmology, 13:S32-S35, 2003.

10. N. Gupta and Y.H. Yücel. Glaucoma and the Brain. Journal of Glaucoma. 10: S28-S29, 2001.

11. Y.H. Yucel, Q. Zhang, L-C Ang, N. Gupta. Evidence for neural degeneration in human glaucoma involving the intracranial optic nerve, lateral geniculate nucleus and visual cortex. Annual Association for Research in Vision and Ophthalmology Meeting, Fort Lauderdale, Florida, April 2004.

12. D.C. Hood and V.C. Greenstein. Multifocal VEP and ganglion cell damage: applications and limitations for the study of glaucoma. Progress in Retinal and Eye Research, 22: 201-251, 2003

13. A. Miki, G. T. Liu, S. A. Englander, et al., Functional magnetic resonance imaging of eye dominance at 4 tesla. Ophthalmic Research, 33276-82, 2001.

Question 8

Should glaucoma patients undergo genetic testing?

Wallace L. M. Alward

It is well established that many forms of glaucoma are heritable.[1] Approximately one-half of patients with primary open angle glaucoma (POAG) have a known family history of glaucoma.[2] The heritable nature of glaucoma has made molecular genetic studies of great interest. It is hoped that through molecular genetic research we will better understand the pathophysiology of glaucoma, develop better therapies for glaucoma, and develop better tests for glaucoma. There has been much progress in glaucoma genetic research. The major genes for glaucoma and glaucoma-related syndromes are listed in the Table. It is easy to imagine a day when genetic testing for glaucoma will be sufficiently sensitive and specific that 40-year-old individuals will undergo a simple blood test that will quantify their risk of ultimately developing glaucoma. Unfortunately, that day has not yet arrived.

I am in the almost unique position of being able to order genetic tests without cost to my patients. Despite this luxury, I rarely find a benefit in ordering routine genetic testing. For POAG there has been only one gene identified, myocilin. While myocilin is very important, it causes only 3-5% of all POAG.[2,3] Additionally, half of adult-onset POAG patients with myocilin mutations have the GLN368Stop mutation. This mutation causes a mild glaucoma that is indistinguishable from ordinary POAG.[4] Identifying patients with this mutation would be intellectually interesting but would not significantly impact the patient's care.

Recently, a test called OcuGene® has become commercially available. The OcuGene® test measures the presence of a polymorphism in the promoter region of the myocilin gene, 1000 base pairs from the beginning of the

35

coding sequence. In a study by Colomb and coworkers on 142 retrospectively selected patients, the presence of this polymorphism was associated a slightly worse visual field score and a worse response to pressure lowering drugs.[5] In 2002 my colleagues and I reported on 393 prospectively recruited POAG patients.[2] We found no influence of the myocilin promoter polymorphism on any measure of glaucoma severity and no value in testing for this sequence variation.

If routine genetic testing is not useful, when is selective genetic testing reasonable? At present, the patients who might benefit from genetic testing are those who have a set of clinical features that match the phenotype of an identified gene. Let me give three examples.

1) If a patient has juvenile onset glaucoma with very high pressures and a very strong family history it would be reasonable to screen this patient for one of the severe mutations in the myocilin gene. If a myocilin mutation was discovered in the family this would allow pre-symptomatic diagnoses of the children and permit careful follow-up to the 50% of offspring who will develop the disease. Equally importantly, it would reassure the 50% without the mutation that they are at no increased risk of developing glaucoma. OcuGene® would not work for this because it does not test for coding sequence mutations. There is a non-profit test available for myocilin mutations. This is done through the Pathology Laboratory at the University of Iowa. Instructions for ordering the test are available at www.carverlab.org.

2) If a patient has many features of a known syndromic form of glaucoma, but the diagnosis is not clear, molecular testing for specific genes may be helpful. For example, I recently sent DNA for testing of the PITX2 and FOXC1 genes on a young boy who has the systemic features of Axenfeld-Rieger syndrome (facial, dental, and umbilical changes), has glaucoma, but does not have the iris hypoplasia or posterior embryotoxon. I felt that knowing his molecular status would give me a better understanding of how these genes work and would give him the opportunity for genetic testing of his offspring once he reaches reproductive age.

3) There is evolving evidence that Axenfeld-Rieger patients with a mutation in the FOXC1 gene may be at risk for also having cardiac valve defects.[6] If further research supports this relationship it may be valuable to test Axenfeld-Rieger patients for mutations in this gene and, if present, refer them for cardiology evaluation.

While I discourage routine glaucoma genetic testing I do want to encourage anyone who cares for a glaucoma family with multiple affected individuals to contact someone interested in molecular genetic research. Families with inherited glaucoma are invaluable and their study may lead to the next major genetic discovery.

In summary, at the present time I cannot recommend routine genetic testing of glaucoma patients. Routine genetic testing is not a cost-effective use of the patient's or society's resources. However, we should all be optimistic that the future for molecular genetic testing is extremely bright.

Gene	Disease
Myocilin	Primary open angle glaucoma (3.3%)[2,3]
	Juvenile open angle glaucoma (6.4%)[2]
	Normal tension glaucoma (1.2%)[2]
	Pigmentary glaucoma (1.5%)[2]
	Exfoliation syndrome (1.7%)[2]
	Ocular Hypertension (2.4%)[2]
Optineurin	Autosomal dominant normal tension glaucoma[7] (a very rare disease)
OPA1	Normal tension glaucoma[8]
CYP1B1	Primary congenital glaucoma[9]
	Peters anomaly
PITX2	Axenfeld-Rieger syndrome[10]
	Peters anomaly
FOXC1	Axenfeld-Rieger syndrome[11]
	Iris hypoplasia
	Peters anomaly
PAX6	Aniridia[12]
	Peters anomaly

This is a partial list and each item is not fully referenced due to space limitations. To research specific genes or diseases the reader is referred to Online Mendelian Inheritance in Man (OMIM): http://www.ncbi.nlm.nih.gov/omim/.

REFERENCES

1. Sheffield VC, Alward WLM, Stone EM. The Glaucomas, 8th ed. In: Scriver CR, Beaudet AL, Sly SS, Valle D, editors. The Metabolic and Molecular Bases of Inherited Disease. New York: McGraw-Hill, 2001.

2. Alward WL, Kwon YH, Khanna CL, et al. Variations in the myocilin gene in patients with open-angle glaucoma. Arch Ophthalmol 2002;120:1189-97.

3. Stone EM, Fingert JH, Alward WLM, et al. Identification of a gene that causes primary open angle glaucoma. Science 1997;275:668-670.

4. Graul TA, Kwon YH, Zimmerman MB, et al. A case-control comparison of the clinical characteristics of glaucoma and ocular hypertensive patients with and without the myocilin Gln368Stop mutation. Am J Ophthalmol 2002;134:884-90.

5. Colomb E, Nguyen TD, Bechetoille A, et al. Association of a single nucleotide polymorphism in the TIGR/MYOCILIN gene promoter with the severity of primary open-angle glaucoma. Clin Genet 2001;60:220-5.

6. Honkanen RA, Nishimura DY, Swiderski RE, et al. A family with Axenfeld-Rieger syndrome and Peters Anomaly caused by a point mutation (Phe112Ser) in the FOXC1 gene. Am J Ophthalmol 2003;135:368-75.

7. Rezaie T, Child A, Hitchings R, et al. Adult-onset primary open-angle glaucoma caused by mutations in optineurin. Science 2002;295:1077-9.

8. Aung T, Ocaka L, Ebenezer ND, et al. A major marker for normal tension glaucoma: association with polymorphisms in the OPA1 gene. Hum Genet 2002;110:52-6.

9. Stoilov I, Akarsu AN, Sarfarazi M. Identification of three different truncating mutations in cytochrome P4501B1 (CYP1B1) as the principal cause of primary congenital glaucoma (Buphthalmos) in families linked to the GLC3A locus on chromosome 2p21. Hum Mol Genet 1997;6:641-7.

10. Semina EV, Reiter R, Leysens NJ, et al. Cloning and characterization of a novel bicoid-related homeobox transcription factor gene, RGS, involved in Rieger syndrome. Nature Genetics 1996;14:392-99.

11. Nishimura DY, Swiderski RE, Alward WLM, et al. The forkhead transcription factor gene FKHL7 is responsible for glaucoma phenotypes which map to 6p25. Nat Genet 1998;19:140-7.

12. Ton CCT, Hirvonen H, Miwa H, et al. Positional cloning and characterization of a paired box- and homeobox-containing gene from the aniridia region. Cell 1991;67:1059-74.

Question 9

What are the ophthalmoscopic signs of glaucomatous optic neuropathy?

Jost B. Jonas

For evaluating the glaucomatous patho-morphology of the optic nerve head, one uses descriptive quantitative and qualitative variables. These are

- size and shape of the optic disc;

- size, shape and pallor of the neuroretinal rim;

- size of the optic cup in relation to the area of the disc;

- configuration and depth of the optic cup;

- cup-to-disc diameter ratio and cup-to-disc area ratio;

- position of the exit of the central retinal vessel trunk on the lamina cribrosa surface;

- presence and location of splinter-shaped hemorrhages;

- occurrence, size, configuration and location of parapapillary chorioretinal atrophy;

- diffuse and/or focal decrease of the diameter of the retinal arterioles; and

- visibility of the retinal nerve fiber layer.

Due to a biologic overlap of almost all quantitative variables between normal subjects and glaucoma patients, qualitative variables such as occurrence of disc hemorrhages and presence of localized retinal nerve fiber layer defects, compared with quantitative variables, have a higher specificity in separating glaucoma eyes from normal eyes

Optic disc size

The importance of the size of the optic disc for diagnosis and pathogenesis of glaucomatous optic neuropathy is based on the finding that the optic disc area shows a marked interindividual variability of about 1:7 in a normal Caucasian population. The optic disc area is independent of age beyond an age of about 3 to 10 years. Caucasians have relatively small optic discs, followed by Mexicans, Asians, and Afro-Americans. In the diagnosis of glaucomatous optic neuropathy, assessment of the optic disc size is of utmost importance since the optic disc size is correlated with the size of the optic cup and neuroretinal rim. A large cup in a large optic disc can, therefore, be normal, while a small optic cup in a very small optic disc suggests glaucomatous optic nerve damage. In glaucoma, the optic disc is normal in size in primary open-angle glaucoma including the juvenile-onset type of primary open-angle glaucoma, the age-related atrophic type of primary open-angle glaucoma, and in secondary open-angle glaucoma due to primary melanin dispersion syndrome ("pigmentary glaucoma"). In all glaucoma eyes with high myopia including the highly myopic type of primary open-angle glaucoma, the optic disc is abnormally large in the sense of secondary macrodiscs acquired due to high myopia.

Neuroretinal rim size

The neuroretinal rim is the intrapapillary equivalent of the retinal nerve fibers and optic nerve fibers. It is, therefore, one of the main targets in the morphologic glaucoma diagnosis. The neuroretinal rim size is correlated with the optic disc area: the larger is the disc, the larger is the rim. The correlation between rim area and disc area corresponds with the positive correlation between optic disc size, optic nerve fiber count, and number and total area of the lamina cribrosa pores. In morphologic glaucoma diagnosis, the neuroretinal rim area is one of the most important quantitative variables. Due to its high interindividual variability in the normal population, however, the overlap between normal subjects and patients with early glaucomatous optic nerve damage is high. This is the disadvantage of many quantitative variables. To achieve a higher diagnostic power, the neuroretinal rim measured in the whole optic disc can be broken up into disc sectors, with the infero-temporal and supero-temporal disc sector having a higher predictive power than the neuroretinal rim as a whole. Reason is the preferential loss of neuroretinal rim in the inferior and superior disc regions in the early to medium advanced stages of the disease.

Neuroretinal rim shape

The neuroretinal rim exhibits a characteristic configuration in normal eyes. It is based on the vertically oval shape of the optic disc and the horizontally oval shape of the optic cup. The neuroretinal rim is usually broadest in the **I**nferior disc region, followed by the **S**uperior disc region, the **N**asal disc area, and finally the **T**emporal disc region (**ISN`T** rule). The characteristic shape of the rim is of utmost importance in the diagnosis of early glaucomatous optic nerve damage in ocular hypertensive eyes prior to the development of visual field defects in white-on-white perimetry.

In glaucoma, neuroretinal rim is lost in all sectors of the optic disc with regional preferences depending on the stage of the disease. In eyes with modest glaucomatous damage, rim loss is found predominantly at the inferotemporal and superotemporal disc regions. In eyes with moderately advanced glaucomatous atrophy, the temporal horizontal disc region is the location with relatively the most marked rim loss. In very advanced glaucoma, the rim remnants are located mainly in the nasal disc sector, with a larger rim portion in the upper nasal region than in the lower nasal region.

In contrast to glaucomatous optic neuropathy, non-glaucomatous optic nerve damage is usually not associated with a loss of neuroretinal rim. Consequently, the shape of the neuroretinal rim is not markedly altered.

Neuroretinal rim pallor

Increasing pallor of the optic disc and especially of the neuroretinal rim is a typical sign of optic nerve damage. The increase in pallor of the neuroretinal rim may be more marked in eyes with non-glaucomatous optic neuropathy than in eyes with glaucoma. In other words, if the neuroretinal rim looks rather pale, the probability for a non-glaucomatous optic neuropathy is higher than for glaucoma. Pallor of the neuroretinal rim is thus one among other variables to differentiate between glaucomatous versus non-glaucomatous optic neuropathy. In glaucoma, the overall pallor of the optic disc as sum of optic cup and neuroretinal rim increases mainly due to the enlargement of the pale optic cup.

Optic cup size in relation to the optic disc size

Also the optic cup shows a high interindividual variability. In normal eyes, the areas of the optic disc and optic cup are correlated with each other: the larger is the optic disc, the larger is the optic cup. In the morphologic diagnosis of glaucoma, this feature has to be taken into account. Early or moderately advanced glaucomatous optic nerve damage may erroneously be overlooked in small optic discs with relatively low cup-to-disc ratios, if one does not take into account that small optic discs normally have no optic cup. The glaucomatous eyes with small optic discs and pseudonormal but glaucomatous minicups often show glaucomatous abnormalities in the parapapillary region such as a decreased visibility of the retinal nerve fiber layer, diffusely and/or focally diminished diameter of the retinal arterioles, and parapapillary chorioretinal atrophy. In contrast, a large optic cup in a large optic disc should not lead to the diagnosis of glaucoma, if the other intrapapillary variables are normal, mainly the configuration of the neuroretinal rim.

In contrast to glaucoma, the optic cup does not markedly enlarge in eyes with non-glaucomatous optic nerve damage. Correspondingly, the neuroretinal rim does not pronouncedly decrease in eyes with non-glaucomatous optic nerve damage. Besides parapapillary atrophy, disc pallor, and depth of the optic cup, the increase in cup area is thus an important marker to differentiate between glaucomatous and non-glaucomatous optic nerve damage.

Cup/disc ratios

The cup/disc ratios in normal eyes are significantly larger horizontally than vertically due to the vertically oval optic disc and the horizontally oval optic cup. In less than 7% of normal eyes the horizontal cup/disc ratio is smaller than the vertical one. It indicates that the quotient of the horizontal-to-vertical-cup/disc ratios is usually higher than 1.0 . This is important for the diagnosis of glaucoma, where, in the early to medium advanced stages, the vertical cup/disc diameter ratio increases faster than the horizontal one.

This leads to a decrease in the quotient of horizontal-to-vertical-cup/disc ratios to values lower than 1.0 . As ratio of cup diameter to disc diameter, the cup/disc ratios depend on the size of the optic disc and cup. The high interindividual variability of the optic disc and cup diameters explains, that the cup/disc ratios range in a normal population between 0.0 and almost 0.9 . Due to the correlation between disc area and cup area, the cup/disc ratios are low in small optic nerve heads, and they are high in large optic discs. An unusually high cup/disc ratio, therefore, can be physiologic in eyes with large optic nerve heads, while an average cup/disk ratio is uncommon in normal eyes with small optic discs. In the diagnosis of glaucomatous optic nerve damage, this interindividual variability of cup/disc ratios and their dependence on the optic disc size has to be taken into account. Eyes with physiologically high cup/disc ratios in macrodiscs should not be overdiagnosed considering them to be glaucomatous, and eyes with increased intraocular pressure, small optic nerve heads, and average or low cup/disc ratios should not be underdiagnosed regarding them to be only "ocular hypertensive". As ratio of cup diameter to disc diameter, the cup/disc ratios are independent of the magnification by the optic media of the examined eye and of the fundus camera or other devices. Methods to correct for the ocular and camera magnification may not have to be applied. The quotient of the horizontal-to-vertical-cup/disc ratios is additionally independent of the size of the optic cup and disc.

Optic disc hemorrhages

Since their description by Drance and Begg in 1970, splinter-shaped or flame-shaped hemorrhages at the border of the optic disc are a hallmark of glaucomatous optic nerve atrophy. Rarely or very rarely found in normal eyes, disc hemorrhages are detected in about 4% to 7% of eyes with glaucoma. Their frequency increases from an early stage of glaucoma to a medium advanced stage and decreases again towards a far advanced stage. One study suggested that disc hemorrhages are not found in disc regions or eyes without detectable neuroretinal rim. In early glaucoma, they are usually located in the inferotemporal or superotemporal disc regions. They are associated with localized retinal nerve fiber layer defects, neuroretinal rim notches and circumscribed perimetrical loss. The diagnostic importance of disc hemorrhages is based on their high specificity, since they are only rarely found in normal eyes; they usually indicate the presence of glaucomatous optic nerve damage even if the visual field is unremarkable; and they suggest progression of glaucoma. Glaucoma, however, is not the only optic nerve disease in which optic disc hemorrhages can be found. In two epidemiological studies, frequency of disc hemorrhages in non-glaucomatous eyes was about 1%. About two months after the initial bleeding, often a localized defect of the retinal nerve fiber layer or a broadening of a localized retinal nerve fiber layer defect can be detected correlating with a circumscribed scotoma in the visual field.

Since frequency of optic disc hemorrhages differs between the various types of the open-angle glaucomas, assessment of disc bleedings can be helpful for classification of the glaucoma type. Disc hemorrhages were found most often in patients with focal normal-pressure glaucoma. Frequency of detected disc bleedings was lower in patients with juvenile-onset primary open-glaucoma, age-related atrophic primary open-angle glaucoma, and highly myopic primary open-angle glaucoma. Disc hemorrhages, however, can be found in all types of the chronic open-angle glaucomas, suggesting that the pathomechanism associated with disc hemorrhages may be present in all these glaucoma types.

Parapapillary chorioretinal atrophy

Ophthalmoscopically, the parapapillary chorioretinal atrophy can be divided into a central beta zone and a peripheral alpha zone. The peripheral zone (alpha zone) is characterized by an irregular hypopigmentation and hyperpigmentation and intimated thinning of the chorioretinal tissue layer. On its outer side it is adjacent to the retina, and on its inner side it is in touch with a zone characterized by visible sclera and visible large choroidal vessels (beta zone), or with the peripapillary scleral ring, respectively. Features of the inner zone (beta zone) are marked atrophy of the retinal pigment epithelium and of the choriocapillaris, good visibility of the large choroidal vessels and the sclera, thinning of the chorioretinal tissues, and round bounds to the adjacent alpha zone on its peripheral side and to the peripapillary scleral ring on its central side. If both zones are present, beta zone is always closer to the optic disc than alpha zone. In indirect and direct clinical-histologic comparisons, beta zone correlates with a complete loss of retinal pigment epithelium cells and a markedly diminished count of retinal photoreceptors. Alpha zone is the equivalent of pigmentary irregularities in the retinal pigment epithelium. Correspondingly, beta zone corresponds psychophysically to an absolute scotoma, and alpha zone to a relative scotoma. In normal eyes, both alpha zone and beta zone are largest and most frequently located in the temporal horizontal sector, followed by the inferior temporal area and the superior temporal region. They are smallest and most rarely found in the nasal parapapillary area. Alpha zone is present in almost all normal eyes and is thus more common than beta zone (mean frequency in normal eyes: about 15%-20%). Alpha zone and beta zone have to be differentiated from the myopic scleral crescent in eyes with high myopia and from the inferior scleral crescent in eyes with "tilted optic discs". The myopic scleral crescent present in highly myopic eyes differs histologically from the glaucomatous beta zone in non-highly myopic eyes. In the region of the myopic crescent, only the inner limiting membrane and underlying retinal nerve fiber layer or its remnants cover the sclera while in the glaucomatous beta zone, Burch's membrane and the choroid is interposed between the remnants of the retina and the sclera. Size, shape and frequency of alpha zone and beta zone do not differ significantly between normal eyes and eyes with nonglaucomatous optic nerve atrophy. Both zones are significantly larger and beta zone occurs more often in eyes with glaucomatous optic nerve atrophy than in normal eyes. Size of both zones and frequency of beta zone are significantly correlated with variables indicating the severity of the glaucomatous optic nerve damage such as neuroretinal rim loss, decrease of retinal vessel diameter, reduced visibility of the retinal nerve fiber bundles, and perimetric defects. A large beta zone, also called "halo glaucomatosus" when encircling the optic disc, is often associated with a marked degree of fundus tessellation, a shallow glaucomatous disc cupping, a relatively low frequency of disc hemorrhages and detectable localized defects of the retinal nerve fiber layer, a mostly concentric loss of neuroretinal rim, and normal or almost normal intraocular pressure measurements. The location of parapapillary chorioretinal atrophy is spatially correlated with the neuroretinal rim loss in the intrapapillary region. It is larger in that sector with the more marked loss of neuroretinal rim.

In contrast to glaucomatous optic neuropathy, non-glaucomatous optic nerve damage does not lead to an enlargement of parapapillary atrophy. It indicates that parapapillary atrophy is one among other optic disc variables to differentiate between glaucomatous versus non-glaucomatous optic nerve damage. Parallel to the spatial association between position of the central retinal vessel trunk and the local loss of neuroretinal in the optic disc, a spatial correlation between the position of the central retinal vessel trunk exit in the lamina cribrosa and the location of parapapillary atrophy has been reported. The longer the distance to the central retinal vessel trunk, the larger is beta zone. The pathogenetic explanation for this finding has remained unclear so far.

Diameter of retinal arterioles

Diffuse narrowing of the retinal vessels has been described for glaucomatous and nonglaucomatous optic neuropathies. In glaucoma, the vessel diameter reduces with decreasing area of the neuroretinal rim, diminishing visibility of the retinal nerve fiber layer, and increasing visual field defects. Since the reduction of the vessel caliber is also found in eyes with nonglaucomatous optic nerve damage such as descending optic nerve atrophy and nonarteritic anterior ischemic optic neuropathy, one inferred that a generalized reduction of the vessel diameter is typical for optic nerve damage but not characteristic for glaucoma. From a pathogenetic point of view, it suggests that vessel reduction is not causative for glaucomatous optic nerve fiber loss but, at least partially, secondary to a reduced demand in the superficial layers of the retina.

Besides diffuse narrowing, the retinal arterioles additionally show focal narrowing of their caliber in eyes with optic nerve damage such as nonarteritic anterior ischemic optic neuropathy and glaucoma. The degree of focal narrowing of the retinal arterioles increased significantly with age in normal eyes. It was significantly higher in eyes with an optic nerve atrophy than in normal eyes. The eyes with glaucoma and the eyes with nonglaucomatous optic nerve damage did not vary significantly in the severity of focal narrowing. Focal arteriole narrowing was slightly more pronounced in eyes with normal-pressure glaucoma and eyes with nonarteritic anterior ischemic optic neuropathy than in the other groups. These differences, however, were not marked. In the glaucoma group, the degree of focal narrowing of the retinal arterioles was significantly more pronounced if the optic nerve damage was more advanced. A recent study comparing fundus photographs and fluorescein angiograms with each other showed that focal narrowing of the retinal arterioles in the parapapillary region of eyes with optic neuropathies represented a real stenosis of the vessel lumen and was not due to an ophthalmoscopic artifact.

Evaluation of the retinal nerve fiber layer

In normal eyes, visibility of the RNFL is regionally unevenly distributed. Dividing the fundus into eight regions, the nerve fiber bundles are most visible in the temporal inferior sector, followed by the temporal superior area, the nasal superior region and finally the nasal inferior sector. It is least visible in the superior, inferior, temporal horizontal and nasal horizontal regions. Correspondingly, the diameters of the retinal arterioles are significantly widest at the temporal inferior disc border, followed the temporal superior disc region, the nasal superior area and finally the nasal inferior disc region. It is in agreement with the location of the foveola below a horizontal line drawn through the center of the optic disc, and with the configuration of the neuroretinal rim that is broadest at the temporal inferior disc border, followed the temporal superior disc region. The sequence of the sectors concerning the best visibility of the RNFL correlates with the sectors' sequence in respect to rim configuration and retinal artery caliber. Visibility of the RNFL decreases with age. This correlates with an age-related reduction of the optic nerve fiber count with an annual loss of about 4,000 to 5,0000 fibers/year out of an original population of approximately 1.4 million optic nerve fibers. These features of the normal RNFL are important for diagnosis of RNFL changes secondary to optic nerve damage in the diseased eye.

Localized defects of the RNFL are defined as wedge-shaped and not spindle-like defects, running towards or touching the optic disc border. If they are pronounced, they can have a broad basis at the temporal raphe of the fundus. Typically occurring in about 20% or more of all glaucoma eyes, they can also be found in eyes with an atrophy of the optic nerve due to other reasons such as optic disc drusen, toxoplasmotic retinochoroidal scars, ischemic retinopathies with cotton-wool spots of the retina, after long-standing papilledema or optic neuritis due to multiple sclerosis, to mention some examples. Since the localized RNFL defects are not present in normal eyes, they almost always signify a pathological abnormality. This is important for subjects with ocular hypertension in which a localized RNFL-defect points to an optic nerve damage even in the absence of perimetric abnormalities. One has to take into account however that localized RNFL defects are not pathognomonic for glaucoma since they occur also in other types of optic nerve atrophy. Due to their relatively low frequency in eyes with an optic nerve damage, their sensitivity to indicate an optic nerve atrophy is not very high. In glaucomatous eyes, the frequency of localized RNFL-defects increases significantly from an "early" glaucoma stage to a stage with medium advanced glaucomatous damage and decreases again to a stage with very marked glaucomatous changes. In eyes with very advanced optic nerve damage they are usually no longer detectable due to the pronounced loss of nerve fibers in all fundus sectors. Localized RNFL defects are detected more often in eyes with the focal type of normal-pressure glaucoma than in eyes with the age-related atrophic type of open-angle glaucoma and the highly myopic type of open-angle glaucoma. In their vicinity at the optic disc border, one often finds notches of the neuroretinal rim, sometimes an optic disc hemorrhage, and a parapapillary chorioretinal atrophy which is relatively more marked in that sector than in other sectors. Localized RNFL-defects are often found six to eight weeks after an optic disc bleeding. They point towards a localized type of optic nerve damage.

With respect to different sectors of the fundus, localized RNFL defects are most often found in the temporal inferior sector followed by the temporal superior sector. In the nasal fundus region, localized RNFL defects are only rarely seen. This may be due to the fact that the RNFL in normal eyes is less detectable in the nasal fundus than in the temporal inferior and temporal superior fundus areas. In fundus areas, in which the RNFL physiologically is thin, also localized defects are harder to be found than in areas with a thick RNFL. It is unclear whether the morphology of the lamina cribrosa with larger pores in the inferior and superior sectors and smaller pores in the temporal and nasal regions plays a role for the development of localized RNFL defects.

The importance of localized defects of the RNFL for the diagnosis of glaucoma have been shown in many studies. Airaksinen described clearly detectable wedge-shaped defects of the RNFL in eyes with increased intraocular pressure and normal visual field. Later, these eyes showed localized perimetric changes when the area of concern was especially examined.

Besides localized RNFL-defects, a diffuse loss of retinal nerve fibers occurs in eyes with a damage of the optic nerve. It leads to a decreased visibility of the RNFL. Ophthalmoscopically, the diffuse RNFL loss is more difficult to detect than a localized defect. It is helpful to use the variable "sequence of fundus sectors concerning the best RNFL visibility". If one detects that in an eye without fundus irregularities the RNFL is markedly better detectable in the temporal superior fundus region than in the temporal inferior sector, it points towards a loss of RNFL mainly in the temporal inferior fundus region. This variable can be examined upon ophthalmoscopy without applying sophisticated techniques. It is also helpful to evaluate whether the retinal vessels are clearly and sharply detectable. The retinal vessels are normally embedded into the RNFL. In eyes with a diffuse RNFL loss, the retinal vessels are covered only by the inner limiting membrane resulting in a better visibility and a sharper image of the large retinal vessels. This is an important variable in the diagnosis of an optic nerve damage.

Considering its great importance in the assessment of anomalies and diseases of the optic nerve and taking into account the feasibility of its ophthalmoscopical evaluation, the retinal nerve fiber layer should be examined during every routine ophthalmoscopy. This holds true especially for patients with an early damage of the optic nerve. The importance to evaluate the RNFL is further exemplified in studies in which a glaucomatous damage of the optic nerve could be detected earlier by examination of the RNFL than by conventional computerized perimetry. It is of utmost importance for the detection of glaucoma in eyes with a pseudonormal but glaucomatous minicup in minidiscs, and it is useful to classify an eye with a pseudoglaucomatous but normal large cup in a large disc as normal. In eyes with advanced optic nerve atrophy, other examination techniques such as perimetry may be more helpful for the follow-up of the optic nerve damage.

REFERENCES

1. Jonas JB, Dichtl A. Evaluation of the retinal nerve fiber layer. Surv Ophthalmol, 1996; 40: 369-378.

2. Jonas JB, Budde WM, Panda-Jonas S. Ophthalmoscopic evaluation of the optic nerve head. Surv Ophthalmol, 1999; 43: 293-320.

3. Jonas JB, Budde WM. Diagnosis and pathogenesis of glaucomatous optic neuropathy: morphological aspects. Progr Retin Eye Res, 2000; 19: 1-40.

Question 10

Is optical coherence tomography useful in the clinical evaluation of glaucoma

Joel S. Schuman

Optical coherence tomography (OCT) can be used to produce high resolution cross-sectional images. It is based on Michelson type interferometry and uses a superluminescent diode in the near infrared wavelength.[1] In the eye this technology may be used in the posterior and anterior segments. The commercial device is in its third generation (StratusOCT, Carl Zeiss Meditec, Inc, Dublin, CA) and has a resolution of approximately 8-10 microns. This discussion will confine itself to the glaucoma applications of OCT.

On the topic of OCT specifically, high resolution non-contact non-invasive cross-sectional imaging may be useful in glaucoma diagnosis and management. The device can create cross-sectional images of the macula, the peripapillary retinal nerve fiber layer and the optic nerve head (Figure 1). By taking a series of radial spoke-like scans centered on the macula, a map is created of macular thickness, identifying areas of edema, atrophy or other abnormalities. Similarly, a series of radial spoke-like scans centered on the optic nerve head produce a topographic optic nerve head map. A 3.4 mm diameter circular scan centered on the optic nerve head produces a cross-sectional image of the retina from which the retinal nerve fiber layer may be directly measured. Glaucoma damage may be measured in the retinal nerve fiber layer, optic nerve head or macula (Figure 2).[2-5]

OCT uses automated algorithms to analyze acquired images. These algorithms do not require user input. The user, however, must assess the quality of the scan prior to analysis, and must evaluate the fit of the analysis

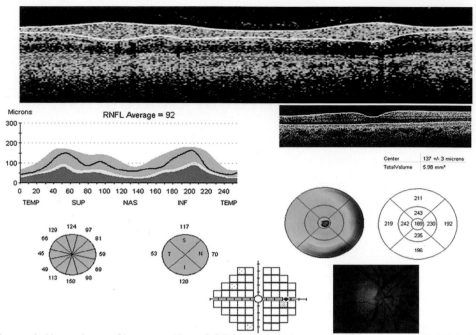

Figure 1. Normal eye. Circumpapillary OCT is shown at upper portion of panel. RNFL is the upper highly reflective layer delimited by white line created by automated algorithm. Below on the left is the quantitative RNFL analysis. In this assessment, green is the 5th -95th percentile by age, yellow is the 1st 5th percentile and red is below the 1st percentile. The data are presented as mean overall, by a-scan (256 a-scans comprise this OCT), by clock hour and by quadrant. To the right is the macular scan and macular map, with quantitative values provided for overall volume, center thickness and for thickness in each of nine sub-areas. The patient optic nerve head photograph and normal Matrix FDT visual field are demonstrated.

to determine whether or not the image was of adequate quality to analyze, and whether or not the algorithm performed properly. A poor image or a poor analysis will result in inaccurate data.

Several groups have now demonstrated the utility of this technology in glaucoma diagnosis. It is at least as good as expert evaluation of stereoscopic optic nerve head photographs, nerve fiber layer photographs, FDT or SWAP in distinguishing normal from glaucomatous eyes.[6,7] OCT evaluation compares favorably to confocal scanning laser ophthalmoscopic optic nerve head evaluation as well as scanning laser polarimetry.[8,9] The fact that OCT is at least as good as expert evaluation of stereoscopic optic nerve head or nerve fiber layer photographs is important for two reasons. First, since the studies used the photographs as the gold standard, OCT

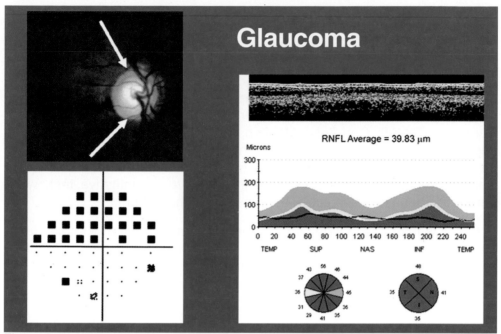

Figure 2. A glaucomatous eye. Upper left shows an optic nerve cupped to the rim inferiorly, and markedly cupped superiorly. Arrows indicate the points of maximal cupping. The visual field corresponds to the neuroretinal rim loss; however, the inferior loss is more questionable, and would likely require repetitive visual fields to confirm. OCT shows thinning of the RNFL both superiorly and inferiorly, confirming the inferior visual field loss, and obviating the need for multiple confirmatory visual field exams. The OCT RNFL loss also is proportional to the field and disc damage, with more loss below than above. This is seen on the quantitative graph showing that the RNFL has dipped further into the abnormal zone inferiorly than superiorly.

could not perform better than photography. Second, if OCT is as good as an expert evaluation of stereoscopic photographs of the optic nerve and nerve fiber layer, then an OCT examination is similar to expert evaluation of a given patient. This standardizes interpretation of ocular structure at an expert level.

Progression detection is a more difficult parameter to evaluate. OCT has been shown to be more sensitive than visual fields in detecting progressive glaucomatous damage[10] however, similar to work with the confocal scanning laser ophthalmoscope, the specificity has not been tested.[11]

It is believed that structural change precedes detectable functional change. Approximately 40% or more of the nerve fiber layer must be lost before functional change can be detected with the gold-standard Swedish Interactive Thresholding Algorithm (SITA, Carl Zeiss Meditec, Inc.) Perimetry. It may be possible to detect more subtle functional loss using more sensitive perimetric techniques, such as frequency doubling technology (FDT, Carl Zeiss Meditec, Inc.) or Short Wavelength Automated Perimetry (SWAP, Carl Zeiss Meditec, Inc.). Even with the more sensitive perimetric techniques, structural imaging may be a means to detect disease early than can be done using current functional measurement techniques. Perhaps more importantly, OCT is an objective, quantitative test, while perimetry requires a subjective response from the patient.

In fact, it is the combination of these tests that may prove most powerful. A subtle visual field defect is often overlooked, and a true defect must be reproducible to be believed. This typically requires multiple visual field tests to confirm the presence of an abnormality or visual field progression. By combining structural and functional testing a visual field abnormality or progression may be validated without the need for repetitive testing. A field defect combined with a corresponding structural abnormality provides a relatively high degree of certainty of the veracity of the abnormality. Conversely, a normal visual field with a normal structural imaging test greatly allays concerns of disease.

REFERENCES

1. Huang D, Swanson EA, Lin CP, et al. Optical coherence tomography. Science, 1991; 254(5035):1178-81.

2. Schuman JS, Hee MR, Puliafito CA, et al. Quantification of nerve fiber layer thickness in normal and glaucomatous eyes using optical coherence tomography. Arch Ophthalmol, 1995;113(5):586-96.

3. Schuman JS, Pedut-Kloizman T, Hertzmark E, et al. Reproducibility of nerve fiber layer thickness measurements using optical coherence tomography. Ophthalmology, 1996; 103(11):1889-98.

4. Guedes V, Schuman JS, Hertzmark E, et al. Optical coherence tomography measurement of macular and nerve fiber layer thickness in normal and glaucomatous human eyes. Ophthalmology, 2003;110(1):177-89.

5. Schuman JS, Wollstein G, Farra T, et al. Comparison of optic nerve head measurements obtained by optical coherence tomography and confocal scanning laser ophthalmoscopy. Am J Ophthalmol, 2003;135(4):504-12.

6. Bowd C, Zangwill LM, Berry CC, et al. Detecting early glaucoma by assessment of retinal nerve fiber layer thickness and visual function. Invest Ophthalmol Vis Sci, 2001; 42(9):1993-2003.

7. Soliman MA, Van Den Berg TJ, Ismaeil AA, et al. Retinal nerve fiber layer analysis: relationship between optical coherence tomography and red-free photography. Am J Ophthalmol, 2002;133(2):187-95.

8. Zangwill LM, Bowd C, Berry CC, et al. Discriminating between normal and glaucomatous eyes using the Heidelberg Retina Tomograph, GDx Nerve Fiber Analyzer, and Optical Coherence Tomograph. Arch Ophthalmol, 2001;119(7):985-93.

9. Bagga H, Greenfield DS, Feuer W, Knighton RW. Scanning laser polarimetry with variable corneal compensation and optical coherence tomography in normal and glaucomatous eyes. Am J Ophthalmol, 2003;135(4):521-9.

10. Wollstein G, Schuman JS, Price LL, Aydin A, Stark PC, Hertzmark E, Lai E, Ishikawa H, Mattox C, Fujimoto JG, Paunescu LA, Optical coherence tomography longitudinal evaluation of retinal thickness in glaucoma. Arch Ophthalmol (In Press).

11. Chauhan BC, McCormick TA, Nicolela MT, LeBlanc RP. Optic disc and visual field changes in a prospective longitudinal study of patients with glaucoma: comparison of scanning laser tomography with conventional perimetry and optic disc photography. Arch Ophthalmol, 2001;119(10):1492-9.

Question 11

Is scanning laser tomography useful in the evaluation of glaucoma?

Balwantray C. Chauhan

Introduction

The two main objectives of examining the optic disc in glaucoma are to (i) determine if the optic disc is normal or glaucomatous and (ii) to determine whether a disc has changed over time. New imaging techniques such as scanning laser tomography (SLT) may enable clinicians to examine more patients and also more frequently compared to more traditional methods such as optic disc photography.

Detection of a glaucomatous optic disc

The ability to objectively detect the presence of a normal or glaucomatous disc depends on the distribution of some quantitative measure (such as cup/disc ratio) in an unselected glaucoma, for example in a population-based screening survey. If the distribution of cup/disc ratios of this population of glaucoma subjects overlaps widely with that of normal subjects then the utility of this parameter is limited. If on the other hand, another parameter were to separate the glaucomatous and non-glaucomatous populations into two distinct groups, then the utility of this parameter is likely to be high. It is widely known that there is a large variation in optic disc size in a normal population,[1] with a ratio of up to 1:7. Since parameters such as cup-disc ratio and neuroretinal rim are positively correlated to disc size, these parameters by themselves have poor sensitivity and specificity for detecting glaucomatous discs.[2] Correcting the rim area for disc size has been suggested as a technique,[3] however its performance in a population-based study has not been tested.

The ability of SLT to distinguish glaucomatous discs from normal ones has been examined by many investigators. The sensitivity and specificity figures of individual indices or combinations of indices using statistical analyses range from 60-95%. Generally speaking, however, the consensus is that used in isolation, SLT may not be adequate for screening purposes.[4] Used in combination with diagnostic tests, however, SLT may be valuable.

Detection of progression

Detection of a change in optic disc appearance should theoretically be less prone to the large inter-individual variability in disc appearance since the changes are always gauged against the variability measurements obtained in the same optic disc. Clearly, however, if the measurements obtained are variable then the ability to detect small changes will be hampered.

With SLT, the automatically computed parameters such as cup-disc ratio, optic disc size, neuroretinal rim and cup volume can be tracked over time for changes. Although one can observe a trend either by studying the raw numbers or graphs of a parameter over time, a formal statistical analysis such as regression can be carried out and a statistical significance of the change over time can be computed. Advantages of this technique include: (i) simplification of a complex set of data into a summary parameter and (ii) use of a clinically meaningful parameter. Disadvantages include: (i) need for a contour line to delineate the disc margin and a reference height for the definition of cupping (ii) a limited number of observations over time, in other words one examination yields only one measurement; (iii) a large number of observations over time may be necessary to determine a meaningful change and (iv) loss of spatial information as a result of obtaining a summary measurement, for example, a focal notch may not be recognised by a summary index.

An alternative approach described recently analyses discrete areas of the whole image acquired (typically the optic disc and peripapillary area).[5] This technique accounts for the inherent variability of measurements within a given localised group of 16 (4 x 4) pixels. An area where there is a steep topographic slope, for example, at the edge of the cup, will have higher variability compared to an located in the flat peripapillary retina. By generating probability maps, the clinician can view the statistical analysis while maintaining the spatial information contained in the image. A comparison of this method with both optic disc photographs judged clinically and with a change of the optic disc parameters has shown it to be sensitive in acute and long-term disc changes.[6] Advantages of this technique include: (i) utilisation of all available data; (ii) preservation of spatial information and (iii) a highly visual technique that is also statistically sound. Disadvantages include: (i) dependence on high quality images; (ii) uncertainty in interpretation (which applies to all new methods).

Conclusion

Modern imaging techniques, such as SLT, have a tremendous potential for use in every day clinical practice. These devices are easy to use, obtain images quickly and in most cases without pupil dilation, and analyse data within seconds. As a result close monitoring of the optic disc, for example at each clinical visit is a real possibility. The most significant potential of SLT is in the detection of change. While at this time, long-term clinical experience is limited, this situation will change in the next few years.

As with any new technique, using this new information clinically will be a challenge. For example, does a small change in the optic disc detected by the probability map analysis translate into clinically significant information? Should a patient's management be altered as a result? Waiting for a confirmation with visual field changes may result in unnecessary delays in changing a patient's management since optic disc changes often preceed visual field changes, particularly early in the disease course. The lack of a "gold standard" is a disadvantage in evaluating new diagnostic techniques in glaucoma. For example, if a visual field change is taken as a gold standard, then optic disc changes which may occur prior to the field changes may be mistaken for false positive findings.

It would be advantageous to use confocal scanning laser tomography to detect changes, however, it would be prudent to carefully examine the optic disc with clinical techniques to confirm these changes. Repeatable progressive changes with scanning laser tomography should be seen as a significant finding.

REFERENCES

1. Jonas JB, Gusek GC, Naumann GO. Optic disc, cup and neuroretinal rim size, configuration and correlations in normal eyes. Invest Ophthalmol Vis Sci, 1988;29:1151-1158.

2. Tielsch JM, Katz J, Singh K, et al. A population-based evaluation of glaucoma screening: the Baltimore Eye Survey. Am J Epidemiol, 1991;134:1102-10.

3. Wollstein G, Garway-Heath DF, Hitchings RA. Identification of early glaucoma cases with the scanning laser ophthalmoscope. Ophthalmology, 1998;105:1557-1563.

4. Ford BA, Artes PH, McCormick TA, et al. Comparison of data analysis tools for detection of glaucoma with the Heidelberg Retina Tomograph. Ophthalmology, 2003; 110:1145-50.

5. Chauhan BC, Blanchard JW, Hamilton DC, LeBlanc RP. Technique for detecting serial topographic changes in the optic disc and peripapillary retina using scanning laser tomography. Invest Ophthalmol Vis Sci, 2000;41:775-82.

6. Chauhan BC, McCormick TA, Nicolela MT, LeBlanc RP. Optic disc and visual field changes in a prospective longitudinal study of patients with glaucoma: comparison of scanning laser tomography with conventional perimetry and optic disc photography. Arch Ophthalmol, 2001;119:1492-9.

Question 12

Is scanning laser polarimetry useful in the clinical evaluation of glaucoma?

Linda Zangwill

Recent improvements in scanning laser polarimetry retinal nerve fiber layer measurements are likely to enhance its usefulness in clinical practice. Identifying retinal nerve fiber layer damage and change is of vital importance for the clinical evaluation of glaucoma. Until recently, evaluation of the RNFL has been subjective, with descriptions of change primarily qualitative. Scanning laser polarimetry provides objective and quantitative measures of the retinal nerve fiber layer (RNFL).

Scanning laser polarimetry analyses the change in the state of polarization, known as retardation, of light that occurs as it passes through birefringent media such as the RNFL. The thicker the birefringent structure, the greater the retardation of transmitted light. Although retardation has been shown to correlate with RNFL thickness,[1] the RNFL is not the only source of birefringence in the eye. The cornea also exhibits birefringence. Until recently, the SLP employed a fixed compensator that assumed all individuals have the same (fixed) corneal retardation. Recent studies have shown that this assumption is incorrect; there is wide variation in the axis and magnitude of corneal polarization, components of corneal retardation, in healthy and glaucoma eyes.[2, 3] In response to these reports, the commercially available SLP has been modified to include a variable corneal polarization compensator (GDx VCC, Laser Diagnostic Technologies, San Diego) to allow compensation for corneal birefringence based on measurements of each individual's eye. A "fixed" corneal compensation assumption is no longer used to extract RNFL retardation from the measured total retardance. Compared to scanning laser polarimetry measurements with fixed corneal compensation, RNFL thickness measurements obtained with the GDX VCC can better discriminate between healthy and glaucoma eyes,[4] and are more strongly associated with visual field indices.[5,6] Furthermore, correction for the axis of corneal polarization reduces the variance of normal retardation measurements.[7]

For a new diagnostic tool to be useful in clinical practice, the measurements should be reproducible, and provide information that has the potential to change management practice so that patients will be better off as a result of the test.[8]

Scanning laser polarimetry with fixed corneal compensation has been shown to be reproducible in clinical settings.[9,10] In addition, as illustrated by the case examples that follow, scanning laser polarimetry provides summary information on the RNFL that, when used with other clinical information can provide a more complete assessment of the clinical status of a patient. In this GDx VCC printout of a healthy eye (Figure 1), all values are within the normal range, and the typical double hump pattern of thicker nerve fiber layer in the superior and inferior regions is apparent on the TSNIT graph. It should be noted that due to the large variation in the number of nerve fibers in the healthy eye, from approximately 750,000 to 1,5 million fibers, RNFL thickness in healthy eyes also varies dramatically, as reflected by the normal range on the TSNIT graph.

In contrast, the GDx VCC printout from this patient with early to moderate glaucoma shows the TSNIT graph depressed in the inferior region (Figure 2, arrows), which corresponds to visual field damage in the superior region. Furthermore, focal RNFL defects are visible in the superior an inferior regions (arrows). To monitor change over time, the GDx provides a serial analysis report that includes color-coded deviation from baseline thickness values for each follow-up examination. Figure 3 shows RNFL thinning over 3 years in a 63-year-old male (arrows). The changes in superior RNFL correspond to increasing visual field damage in the inferior region during the same follow-up period.

It is important to note that the compensation for corneal retardation should be reassessed after corneal laser refractive procedures or other conditions that may cause a change the corneal architecture. Recent studies have shown LASIK can cause a measurable change in corneal retardation in some eyes.[11,12] In addition, as corneal retardation is neutralized based on macular measurements of Henle's layer, macula pathologies can influence

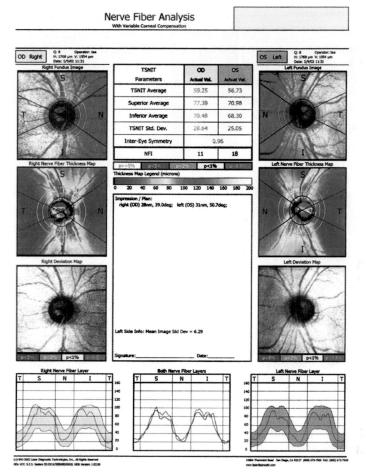

Figure 1. GDx VCC printout from a 35-year-old male shows the fundus image, RNFL parameters, retardation or thickness map, deviation (from normal values) map, and TSNIT graph. All values are within the normal range. In addition, the printout provides a neural network derived number, the "Nerve Fiber Indicator" reflecting the probability that an eye has glaucoma. The NFI is low (17 OD and 18 OS) indicating a low probability that the eye has glaucoma.

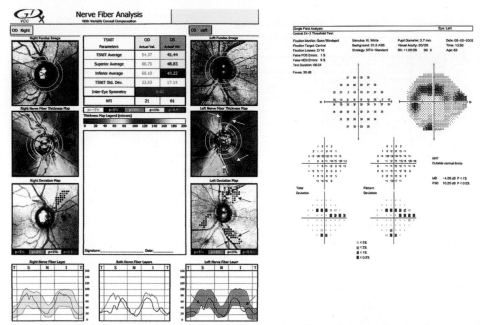

Figure 2. GDx VCC printout from a 64-year-old female with early to moderate glaucoma (visual field mean deviation = -4.08 dB) in the left eye. The inferior RNFL thinning corresponds to superior visual field damage (arrows). In contrast to measurements of the right eye, several of the GDX RNFL measurements of the left eye are outside of the normal range and focal defects are visible in the superior and inferior regions (arrows).

the ability to adequately compensate for corneal retardation in some patients.[13] Alternative techniques to effectively compensate for corneal retardation are under investigation.[13]

In summary, scanning laser polarimetry provides objective and quantitative measures of the retinal nerve fiber layer (RNFL). It often can assist the clinician in diagnosing glaucoma, and shows potential for assessing progression.

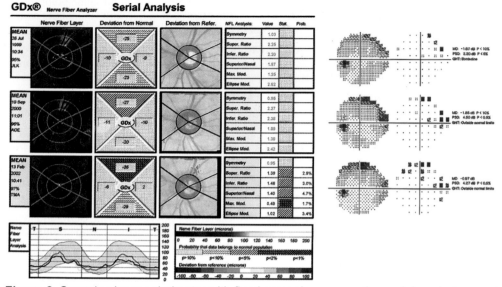

Figure 3. Scanning laser polarimetry with fixed corneal compensation serial analysis report of a 63-year-old male glaucoma patient depicting progressive RNFL thinning over 3 years. The changes in superior RNFL correspond to increasing visual field damage in the inferior region during the same follow-up period. The GDx scans and visual fields were obtained on the same days.

REFERENCES

1. Weinreb RN, Dreher AW, Coleman A, Quigley H, Shaw B, Reiter K. Histopathologic validation of Fourier-ellipsometry measurements of retinal nerve fiber layer thickness. Arch Ophthalmol, 1990;108:557-60.

2. Weinreb RN, Bowd C, Greenfield DS, Zangwill LM. Measurement of the magnitude and axis of corneal polarization with scanning laser polarimetry. Arch Ophthalmol, 2002; 120:901-6.

3. Greenfield DS, Knighton RW, Huang XR. Effect of corneal polarization axis on assessment of retinal nerve fiber layer thickness by scanning laser polarimetry. Am J Ophthalmol, 2000;129:715-22.

4. Weinreb RN, Bowd C, Zangwill LM. Glaucoma detection using scanning laser polarimetry with variable corneal polarization compensation. Arch Ophthalmol, 2003; 121:218-24.

5. Bagga H, Greenfield DS, Feuer W, Knighton RW. Scanning laser polarimetry with variable corneal compensation and optical coherence tomography in normal and glaucomatous eyes. Am J Ophthalmol, 2003;135:521-9.

6. Bowd C, Zangwill LM, Weinreb RN. Association between scanning laser polarimetry measurements using variable corneal polarization compensation and visual field sensitivity in glaucomatous eyes. Arch Ophthalmol, 2003;121:961-6.

7. Greenfield DS, Knighton RW, Feuer WJ, Schiffman JC. Normative retardation data corrected for the corneal polarization axis with scanning laser polarimetry. Ophthalmic Surg Lasers Imaging, 2003;34:165-71.

8. Jaeschke R, Guyatt G, Lijmer J. Diagnostic Tests. In: Guyatt G, Rennie D, eds. Users' Guides to the Medical Literature. Essentials of Evidence-Based Clinical Practice. Chicago: AMA Press, 2002:187-217.

9. Colen TP, Tjon-Fo-sang MJ, Mulder PG, Lemij HG. Reproducibility of measurements with the nerve fiber analyzer (NFA/GDx). J Glaucoma, 2000;9:363-70.

10. Zangwill L, Berry CA, Garden VS, Weinreb RN. Reproducibility of retardation measurements with the nerve fiber analyzer II. J Glaucoma, 1997;6:384-9.

11. Zangwill LM, Abunto T, Bowd C, Angeles R, Schanzlin D, Weinreb RN. Scanning laser polarimetry retinal nerve fiber layer thickness measurements after assisted in Situ Keratomieusis (LASIK). Amer J Ophthalmol 2005 (in press).

12. Angeles R, Abunto T, Bowd C, Zangwill LM, Schanzlin D, Weinreb RN. Corneal changes after laser in situ keratomileusis: measurement of corneal polarization and magnitude and axis. Am J Ophthalmol 2004;137:697-703.

13. Bagga H, Greenfield DS, Knighton RW. Scanning laser polarimetry with variable corneal compensation: identification and correction for corneal birefringence in eyes with macular disease. Invest Ophthalmol Vis Sci, 2003;44:1969-76.

Question 13

Is frequency doubling technology (FDT) perimetry useful in the clinical evaluation of glaucoma?

Philip P. Chen

Frequency doubling technology (FDT) perimetry (Zeiss Meditec, Dublin, California, USA) uses the frequency doubling illusion to detect glaucomatous damage by uncovering functional defects in the relatively small population of magnocellular cells.[1-4] Kelly[1] demonstrated this phenomenon, which occurs when a low spatial frequency (0.25 cycles/degree) sinusoidal grating undergoes rapid (25 Hz) counterphase flicker.

FDT has two principal modes: a full-threshold test that takes approximately 5 minutes to complete, and a screening mode that takes one minute per eye.[5] FDT tests the central 20 degrees around fixation, divided into a grid of 17 locations, comprised of one location at fixation, four locations surrounding fixation, and 12 peripheral locations. An algorithm that also tests an extra 10 degrees nasally can be used. FDT in both the screening and full threshold modes has been shown to be useful in detection of glaucoma, with generally high specificity (85-100%) and high sensitivity (78-100%) for glaucomatous visual field defects seen on standard automated perimetry (SAP).[5] As with other modes of perimetry, learning effect is seen with FDT.[6,7]

Several longitudinal studies have examined the utility of FDT for detection of glaucoma progression. Bayer and Erb[8] described the use of FDT along with Short Wavelength Automated Perimetry and pattern electroretinography in 152 POAG patients followed for 30 months. Using criteria for progression from the Collaborative Normal Tension Glaucoma Study, 54 eyes showed progression on SAP, and 40 of these eyes (74%) showed FDT defects before SAP progression was seen. Notably, among 84 eyes that did not show progression on SAP, 36% had progressive defects on FDT (35% with SWAP).

Joson et al.[9] described a group of 102 eyes of 73 patients who had taken C-20-1 screening FDT, including patients with glaucoma, ocular hypertensives, and glaucoma suspects. Defects seen on FDT were compared with the corresponding locations on initial and subsequent SAP, with a defect at the SAP location defined as at least 50% of the points abnormal (P < .05 on the total deviation plot). Of 279 total locations with FDT defects, 192 (69%) corresponding defects were seen on initial SAP. After an average of 38 months of follow up, this had increased to 216 (77%) defects on final SAP. Fifty two locations with FDT defect never developed a defect on SAP.

Landers et al.[10] prospectively studied 62 patients with ocular hypertension and normal SAP, who had C-20 full threshold FDT and SAP yearly. Five developed SAP defects over a 3 year follow up, and all had FDT defects that preceded development of SAP defects by 27 months (median). Another 5 had FDT defects and did not develop SAP defects during the study.

Medeiros et al.[11] prospectively studied 105 patients (ocular hypertensives or with pre-perimetric glaucoma) with SAP and C-20 and N-30 full threshold FDT. They found 17 developed SAP progression during follow up of 41 months, of which 10 (59%) showed FDT abnormalities before SAP defects, up to 4 years earlier. Four subjects had FDT abnormalities after SAP progression had occurred, and 3 did not show repeatable FDT abnormalities during follow up. FDT defects were signficantly associated with SAP progression (Hazard Ratio = 3.68, P = .04). Among 88 subjects without SAP progression, 21 (24%) had repeatable abnormalities.

Anderson and Johnson have noted the relatively large stimulus size (10 degrees) to be a limitation of current FDT for monitoring glaucoma.[5] Research using a 4 degree stimulus has shown that characteristics of FDT perimetry which might make it more useful than SAP for discerning progression, such as low intra- and intertest fluctuation, are maintained with the smaller stimulus size.[12] Future studies may show FDT to be better than SAP for clinical evaluation of glaucoma.

REFERENCES

1. Kelly DH. Frequency doubling in visual responses. J Opt Soc Am 1966;56:1628-33.

2. Quigley HA, Dunkelberger GR, Green WR. Chronic human glaucoma causing selectively greater loss of large optic nerve fibers. Ophthalmology 1988;95:357-63.

3. Quigley HA, Sanchez RM, Dunkelberger GR, et al. Chronic glaucoma selectively damages large optic nerve fibers. Invest Ophthalmol Vis Sci 1987;28:913-18.

4. Maddess T, Henry GH. Performance of nonlinear visual units in ocular hypertension and glaucoma. Clin Vision Sci 1992;7:371-83.

5. Anderson AJ, Johnson CA. Frequency-doubling technology perimetry. Ophthalmol Clin N Am 2003;16:213-225.

6. Iester M, Capris P, Pandolfo A, Zingirian M, Traverso CE. Learning effect, short-term fluctuation, and long-term fluctuation in frequency doubling technique. Am J Ophthalmol 2000;130:160-164.

7. Joson PJ, Kamantigue MEG, Chen PP. Learning effects among perimetric novices in Frequency Doubling Technology perimetry. Ophthalmology 2002;109:757-60.

8. Bayer AU, Erb C. Short wavelength automated perimetry, frequency doubling technology perimetry, and pattern electroretinography for prediction of progressive glaucomatous standard visual field defects. Ophthalmology 2002;109:1009-17.

9. Joson PJ, Kamantigue MEG, Chen PP. Predictive value of frequency doubling technology perimetry for visual field defects in standard automated perimetry. Poster presentation at the annual meeting of the American Academy of Ophthalmology, Orlando, Florida, U.S.A., October 2002.

10. Landers JA, Goldberg I, Graham SL. Detection of early visual field loss in glaucoma using frequency-doubling perimetry and short-wavelength automated perimetry. Arch Ophthalmol. 2003;121:1705-10.

11. Medeiros FA, Sample PA, Weinreb RN. Frequency doubling technology perimetry abnormalities as predictors of glaucomatous visual field loss. Am J Ophthalmol. 2004;137:863-71.

12. Johnson CA, Cioffi GA, Van Buskirk EM. Frequency doubling technology using a 24-2 stimulus presentation pattern. Optom Vis Sci 1999;76:571-81.

Question 14

Is SWAP useful in the clinical evaluation of glaucoma?

Christopher A. Girkin

Introduction

The development of specialized methods of perimetry involved modifying visual field stimuli to fit the maximal response characteristics of different retino-genticulate ganglion cell populations. Short-wavelength automated perimetry (SWAP) uses a blue stimulus presented against a yellow background and is designed to emphasize the response characteristics of the koniocellular system that conveys information concern blue-yellow color opponency.

Early clinical studies demonstrating tritan-like deficits on tests evaluating foveal function in glaucoma stimulated researchers to develop a test to evaluate this short-wavelength system in the retinal periphery. A standard perimeter was modified to project a 440-nm narrow band size V blue stimulus presented against a broad band 500-700 nm yellow background for 200-msec to maximize spatial and temporal summation, further enhancing isolation of the short-wavelength sensitive pathway.[1]

Currently, SWAP is the most rigorously evaluated specialized perimetric technique, and several clinical studies have been performed with SWAP that illustrate the tests strengths and weakness in the assessment of functional deficits in glaucoma. SWAP defects have been shown to correlate with structural changes of the optic disc and peripapillary retina consistent with glaucoma.[2] SWAP also compares favorably to SAP in the correlation to topographic measurements of the optic disc obtained with confocal scanning laser ophthalmoscopy with mean deviation of SWAP

71

demonstrating an equal or higher degree of correlation, depending on which optic disc parameter was used.[3]

Additionally, two independent studies aimed at evaluating SWAP in early detection have demonstrated the value of SWAP in the detection of visual defects that precede defect on standard perimetry by 3 to 5 years.[4,5] SWAP defects occur in 15 to 30% of patients with ocular hypertension with normal visual fields by standard perimetry, and correlates with the level of risk categorization in these patients.[4] Furthermore, SWAP defects are more extensive than defects on SAP in most subjects with glaucomatous visual field loss.[6] In the OHTS study, while there was a higher prevalence of SWAP defects, the incidence of the development of new SWAP defects was equivalent to that of SAP, indicating that these two techniques are measuring similar disease processes. Additionally, progression using SWAP corresponds to progression of the optic disc defined by masked stereophoto graders to a higher degree that standard perimetry (Figures 1 and 2).[7]

While the initially studies using SWAP demonstrating an enhanced sensitivity to the detection of early glaucomatous damage, SWAP has several limitations. SWAP has shown a higher intertest variability and is more dramatically effected by cataractous change than standard achromatic perimetry.[8] Despite this higher variability, SWAP has been shown to detect progression at a similar rate to standard achromatic perimetry, possible due to its improved sensitivity.[9] Using the pattern deviation plots may help in the interpretation of SWAP visual field defects in patients with significant media opacities.[10] Additionally, the generalized use of SWAP is limited due to the prolonged testing time associated with this technique. Testing time usually ranges from 12-15 minutes and the stimulus is more difficult to determine onset and offset due to the slower response characteristics of the koniocellular ganglion cells, which adversely affects patients acceptance and fatigue.

These limitations with SWAP have prompted researchers to develop SITA algorithms for SWAP testing which may help reduce both testing time and threshold variability. This technique has been effective at decreasing testing time with standard visual field testing and has dramatically reduced the testing time with SWAP to under four minutes in many patients. However, clinical studies to further define the role of SITA-SWAP in clinical management of glaucoma patients are in their early stages.

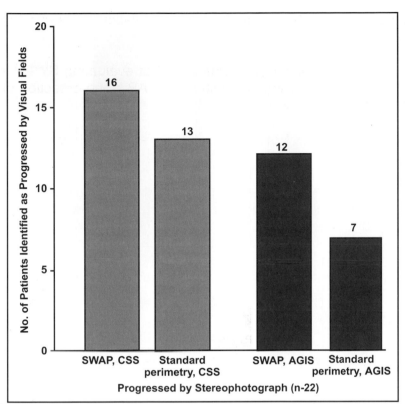

Figure 1. Number of patients with progressive optic disc cupping found to have progressed using visual fields. SWAP indicates short-wavelength automated perimetry; CSS, clinical scoring system; and AGIS, Advanced Glaucoma Intervention Study Criteria.

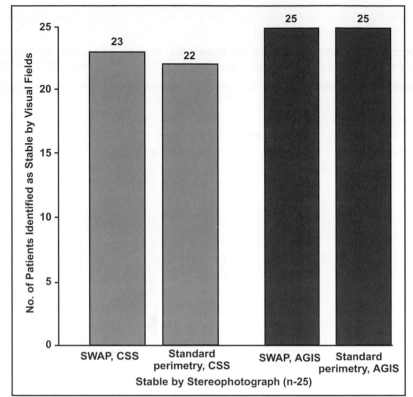

Figure 2. Number of patients with stable optic discs found stable using visual fields. SWAP indicates short-wavelength automated perimetry; CSS, clinical scoring system; and AGIS, Advanced Glaucoma Intervention Study Criteria.

REFERENCES

1. Sample PA, Johnson CA, Haegerstrom-Portnoy G, Adams AJ. Optimum parameters for short-wavelength automated perimetry. J Glaucoma. 1996;5:375-83.

2. Larrosa JM, Polo V, Pablo L, Pinilla I, Fernandez FJ, Honrubia FM. Short-wavelength automated perimetry and neuroretinal rim area. Eur J Ophthalmol. 2000;10:116-20.

3. Teesalu P, Vihanninjoki K, Airaksinen PJ, Tuulonen A, Laara E. Correlation of blue-on-yellow visual fields with scanning confocal laser optic disc measurements. Invest Ophthalmol Vis Sci. 1997;38:2452-9.

4. Sample PA, Taylor JD, Martinez GA, Lusky M, Weinreb RN. Short-wavelength color visual fields in glaucoma suspects at risk. Am J Ophthalmol. 1993;115:225-33.

5. Johnson CA, Adams AJ, Casson EJ, Brandt JD. Blue-on-yellow perimetry can predict the development of glaucomatous visual field loss. Arch Ophthalmol. 1993;111:645-50.

6. Sample PA, Weinreb RN. Color perimetry for assessment of primary open-angle glaucoma. Invest Ophthalmol Vis Sci. 1990;31:1869-75.

7. Girkin CA, Emdadi, A, Blumenthal EZ, Sample PA, Zangwill L, Weinreb RN.Correlation of short wavelength automated perimetry and white-on-white perimetry with progressive optic nerve cupping. Archives of Ophthalmology. 118:1231-6, 2000.

8. Wild JM. Short wavelength automated perimetry. Acta Ophthalmol Scand. 2001; 79:546-59.

9. Johnson CA, Adams AJ, Casson EJ, Brandt JD. Progression of early glaucomatous visual field loss as detected by blue- on-yellow and standard white-on-white automated perimetry. Arch Ophthalmol. 1993;111:651-6.

10. Sample PA, Martinez GA, Weinreb RN. Short-wavelength automated perimetry without lens density testing. American Journal of Ophthalmology. 1994;118:632-41.

Question 15

When should UBM be performed in the evaluation of glaucoma?

Celso Tello

Ultrasound biomicroscopy (UBM, Paradigm Medical Industries, Inc., Salt Lake City, Utah) is a non-invasive diagnostic technique that uses high frequency transducers to provide high resolution, *in vivo* imaging of the anterior segment.[1,2] The currently available commercial unit operates at 50 MHz and provides lateral and axial resolution of approximately 50 µm and 25 µm, respectively. Tissue penetration is approximately 4 to 5 mm. The technique of performing UBM has been reported in detail elsewhere and is similar to traditional immersion B-scan ultrasonography.[1-4]

Angle-closure glaucomas are characterized by mechanical blockage of the trabecular meshwork by the peripheral iris. This alteration in anterior segment anatomy can be caused by changes in the relative or absolute sizes or positions of anterior segment structures or by forces originating in the anterior or posterior segments. UBM is capable of imaging the anterior chamber angle and the structures behind the iris, which is helpful to clarify the underlying mechanisms of the different forms of ACG and assist in management. UBM can help differentiate the angle closure glaucomas due to: pupillary block, plateau iris, phacomorphic glaucoma, and aqueous misdirection or malignant glaucoma.[5]

Pupillary block is the most common form of angle-closure glaucoma. In this condition flow of aqueous from the posterior chamber, to the anterior chamber, is limited by resistance through the pupil at the level of iridolenticular contact. The accumulation of aqueous in the posterior chamber forces the peripheral iris anteriorly, causing anterior iris bowing, narrowing of the angle, and acute or chronic angle-closure glaucoma. UBM can document the iris bowing, the occlusion of the trabecular meshwork by the peripheral iris and the increased volume of the posterior chamber (Figure 1 A). Laser iridotomy equalizes pressure between the anterior chamber and posterior chamber opening the anterior chamber angle and flattening the iris as demonstrated by UBM (Figure 1 B).

In plateau iris, a large or anteriorly positioned ciliary body mechanically holds the peripheral iris against the trabecular meshwork. UBM is the only available technology that can image the ciliary body *in vivo* and it has been instrumental for understanding the pathophysioly of this condition.[2]

In pseudoplateau iris the anterior displacement of the peripheral iris is most commonly caused by cysts of the iris and or ciliary body neuroepithelium,[6] UBM can be very useful for making this diagnosis.

In phacomorphic angle closure abnormalities in the size or position of the lens can alter the anatomic relationship of the anterior segment structures leading to angle-closure glaucoma.

UBM has allowed us to identify at least 2 distinct mechanisms that may be responsible for what is usually called postoperative malignant glaucoma. In the first group, the ciliary body is detached and rotated anteriorly causing angle-closure (Figure 2 A). In the second group the anterior chamber angle is closed but the ciliary body is not detached or anterioly rotated (Figure 2 B). It

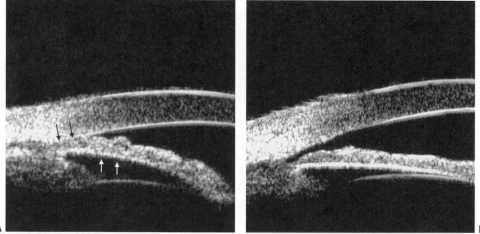

A   B

Figs. 1 A e B – (A) Pupillary block angle-closure, is characterized by a convex iris configuration (white arrows). The angle is closed (black arrows). (B). Laser iridotomy, allows aqueous access to the anterior chamber and the pressure gradient is eliminated. The iris assumes a flat (planar) configuration and the angle opens.

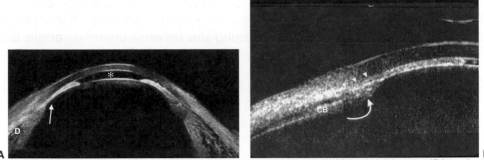

Figs. 2 A e B – (A) Malignant glaucoma caused by ciliary body (CB) detachment (D) and anterior rotation. The anterior chamber (asterisk) is flat and the lens-iris diaphragm (arrow) is rotated forward causing mechanical angle-closure. (B). Aqueous misdirection with absence of ciliary body (CB) detachment. The anterior chamber (asterisk) is flat and the lens-iris diaphragm (curved arrow) is rotated forward causing mechanical angle-closure. (white arrowheads).

is possible that in this group of patients a true misdirection of aqueous to the vitreous cavity occurs increasing the posterior segment pressure which forces the lens and iris against the trabecular meshwork.[7,8]

UBM has helped us better understand the pathophysiology of pigment dispersion syndrome and pigmentary glaucoma.[9,10] In clinical practice, UBM is used to document the iris concavity and the amount of iridozonular contact. Flattening of the iris and relieved of the iridozonular contact can be seen with UBM after miotic treatment or laser iridotomy.

Ocular trauma may result in diverse anterior segment pathologies including hyphema, iridodialysis, cyclodialysis, and angle recession, among others that may cause glaucoma. UBM is useful to detect and differentiate these anatomical changes. Another use includes evaluation of the anterior segment configuration in patients with opaque media such as Peter's anomaly, sclerocornea and congenital glaucoma. By imaging the architecture of a trabeculectomy and localizing the anatomical levels of blockage in failing or failed filtering procedures UBM can assist in the surgical management.

REFERENCES

1. Pavlin CJ, Harasiewicz K, Sherar MD, et al. Clinical use of ultrasound biomicroscopy. Ophthalmology, 1991;98:287-295.

2. Pavlin CJ, Harasiewicz K, Eng P, et al. Ultrasound biomicroscopy of anterior segment structures in normal and glaucomatous eyes. Am J Ophthalmol 1992;113:381-389.

3. Tello C, Liebmann J, Potash SD, et al. Measurement of ultrasound biomicroscopy images: intraobserver and interobserver reliaility. Invest Ophthalmol Vis Sci 1994; 35:3549-3553.

4. Tello C, Liebmann JM, Ritch R. An improved coupling medium for ultrasound biomicroscopy. Ophthalmic Surg 1994;25:410-411.

5. Ritch R, Liebmann J, Tello C. A construct for understanding angle-closure glaucoma: the role of ultrasound biomicroscopy. Ophthalmol Clin N Amer 1995;8:281-293.

6. Azuara-Blanco A, Spaeth GL, Araujo SV, et al. Plateau iris syndrome associated with multiple ciliary body cysts. Report of three cases. Arch Ophthalmol 1996;114:666-668.

7. Liebmann JM, Weinreb RN, Ritch R. Angle-closure glaucoma associated with occult annular ciliary body detachment. Arch Ophthalmol 1998;116:731-755.

8. Tello C, Chi T, Shepps G, et al. Ultrasound biomicroscopy in pseudophakic malignant glaucoma. Ophthalmology 1993;100:1330-1334.

9. Potash SD, Tello C, Liebmann J, et al. Ultrasound biomicroscopy in pigment dispersion syndrome. Ophthalmology 1994;101:332-339.

10. Liebmann JM, Tello C, Chew S-J, et al. Prevention of blinking alters iris configuration in pigment dispersion syndrome and in normal eyes. Ophthalmology 1995;102:446-455.

Question 16

Are there methods for assessing ocular blood flow in clinical practice that are relevant to glaucoma diagnosis and management?

George A. Cioffi

In recent years, there have been many publications examining the relationship between the circulation of the eye and glaucoma. It is believed that circulatory abnormalities occur in greater frequency in individuals with glaucoma and that vascular insufficiency leads to the development of glaucomatous optic neuropathy. Most of these studies hypothesize that vascular perfusion of the optic nerve or retina can be measured and that ischemia within these tissues leads to retinal ganglion cell death. Therefore it is natural to ask the question; Are there methods for assessing ocular blood flow in clinical practice that are relevant to glaucoma diagnosis and management?

There are many important unanswered questions regarding research into the relationship between ocular blood flow and glaucoma. Before attempting to clinically assess the ocular hemodynamics, one must remember that there are a series of sequential assumptions upon which all "glaucoma blood flow" studies are based.

The three assumptions[1,2] are: 1) optic nerve ischemia directly causes or increases the susceptibility of the optic nerve to glaucomatous damage, 2) the present knowledge of the optic nerve vascular anatomy and physiology allows investigators to identify the vascular beds of importance in this neuropathy, and 3) current measurement techniques provide the ability to monitor these vascular beds. The vascular hypothesis of glaucoma is based upon these three critically important, but unproven assumptions.[1,2]

Abnormalities in the circulation to the anterior optic nerve have been cited by many investigators, as a potential causative factor in the development of glaucomatous optic neuropathy.[3-5] There are many clinical reasons to believe that microvascular factors are important. However, many of these studies remain controversial, as the validity of the various hemodynamic measurement techniques remains under investigation. While the hypothesis that circulatory abnormalities are related to the development of glaucomatous optic neuropathy is well supported by clinical associations, this hypothesis remains to be proven. The direct evidence that ischemia is related to glaucoma, as a causative factor, is still lacking.

The second assumption relates specifically to the anatomy and physiology of the ocular vasculature. If we wish to monitor circulatory aberrations in the eye that are associated with the development of glaucoma, our understanding of vascular anatomy and physiology must be sufficient to tell us where to look. The coexistence of glaucomatous optic nerve damage and anatomic/physiologic abnormalities has been offered as potential proof of a casual relationship.[2,3,5,6] Yet causality remains difficult to prove without longitudinal studies. Although our understanding of the ocular vasculature has increased, we still need to have a better understanding of the ocular vascular anatomy. We also need to enhance our understanding of the complex regulatory system, which governs optic nerve, retinal and choroidal perfusion.

The final assumption is that current investigative techniques provide reliable and accurate information about the circulatory status of the optic nerve. If we accept that ischemia is related to the development of glaucomatous optic neuropathy and we establish which vascular beds are important in glaucoma, do current measurement techniques provide the necessary tools for the assessment of these vascular beds?

Non-invasive monitoring of ocular blood flow in humans remains a technology in need of validation. Over the past several decades, many highly technical methods have been developed to examine in vivo ocular hemodynamics, but the validity of each of these methods has not been fully demonstrated.[7,8] This has limited the clinical usefulness of these tests. Failure to validate these technologies has also lead to a conceptual stagnation, as un-supportable conclusions have confused our understanding of the relationship between blood flow and glaucoma. These technologies include Doppler ultrasound, laser Doppler flowmetry, and scanning laser angiography. The various imaging techniques allow us to assess the retrobulbar and intraocular hemodynamics. However, limitations, such as the Doppler techniques' measurement of only blood flow velocity and fluorescein techniques' relatively low resolution, have constrained their usefulness.

Only with validation of these machines will we better understand ocular hemodynamics in health and disease. Deciphering the myriad of numerical values produced by these instruments has become a daunting task. In a recent article, Hayreh examined the scope of these techniques, and elucidated questions of validity, reproducibility, variability, accuracy, confounding agents, and clinical pertinence which still exist.[8] Presently, there is no single method to assess the circulatory status of the human eye, and familiarity with the technique in question is always necessary to interpret the resulting data. The wise clinician cautiously awaits better validation of these technologies before basing therapeutic decision upon them.

REFERENCES

1. Cioffi GA. "Three Common Assumptions About Ocular Blood Flow and Glaucoma". Surv of Ophth Vol 45, Supplement, May 2001, S325-330.

2. Cioffi GA, Wang L. Optic nerve blood flow in glaucoma. Semin Ophthalmol, 1999; 14(3);164-70.

3. Van Buskirk EM, Cioffi GA. Glaucomatous optic neuropathy. Am J Ophthalmol, 1992; 113:447-452.

4. Flammer J. The vascular concept of glaucoma. Surv Ophthalmol, 1994;38:S3-6 .

5. Hayreh SS. Progress in the understanding of the vascular etiology of glaucoma. Curr Opin Ophthalmol, 1994;5:26-35.

6. Yin ZQ, Vaegan, Millar TJ, Beaumont P, Sarks S. Widespread choroidal insufficiency in primary open-angle glaucoma. J Glaucoma, 1997;6:23-32 .

7. Harris A, Kagemann L, Cioffi GA. Assessment of human ocular hemodynamics. Surv Ophthalmol, 1998;42:509-533.

8. Hayreh SS. Evaluation of optic nerve head circulation: review of the methods used. J Glaucoma, 1997;6:319-330.

Question 17

What is the earliest detectable sign of glaucoma?

Jost B. Jonas

The earliest detectable morphologic sign in glaucoma markedly depends on the normal appearance of the individual optic nerve head. Features of normal optic nerve heads are the physiologic neuroretinal rim shape following the ISNT rule, and the relationship between cup size and disc size in small discs. The ISNT rule describes the normal rim shape being usually widest at the inferior disc pole, followed by the superior disc pole, the nasal disc region, and finally the temporal disc region. In an optic disc with an optic cup, rim shape (ISNT-rule) is an important parameter for the early diagnosis of glaucoma. The relationship between cup size and disc size in small discs describes that small optic discs normally do not show cupping, and that large optic discs physiologically have a primary macro-cup. Additional signs for normality are a good visibility of the retinal nerve fiber layer, which usually is slightly better detectable in the temporal inferior region, followed by the temporal superior region, the nasal superior region, and finally the nasal inferior region.

For the early detection of glaucoma, several morphologic parameters are important depending on the size and shape of the optic disc itself. These optic disc variables can be divided into qualitative parameters and quantitative parameters. Qualitative parameters assessable by simple ophthalmoscopy are an abnormal neuroretinal rim shape not following the ISNT rule, i.e. the rim width is more or less equal or smaller at the inferior disc pole and / or superior disc pole compared to the temporal disc region; presence of flame-shaped hemorrhages inside of the disc or touching the disc border; and presence of localized retinal nerve fiber layer defects. For these qualitative parameters, the specificity is high since they usually do not occur in normal eyes. Among the qualitative parameters, sensitivity may be highest for the neuroretinal rim shape (ISNT-rule) showing that assessment of the rim shape in eyes with disc cupping is of utmost importance for the early detection of glaucoma. Assessment of the presence of beta zone of parapapillary atrophy as a qualitative parameter is also helpful for the detection of glaucoma and for differentiating the various phenotypes of the chronic open-angle glaucomas. Due to its relatively high frequency in normal eyes (about 25%), beta zone is, however, a variable of lower diagnostic precision in detecting early glaucomatous abnormalities.

Quantitative parameters have to be examined by measuring techniques, such as confocal laser scanning tomography, planimetry of optic disc photographs, and retinal nerve fiber layer polarimetry. As with any quantitative biologic parameter, optic disc variables have a pronounced interindividual variability; therefore, there is a marked overlap between normality and early glaucoma. Quantitative features of glaucomatous discs are an abnormally small neuroretinal rim related to disc size; cup/disc diameter ratios being vertically higher than horizontally reflecting that the ISNT rule is not fulfilled; an optic cup being too large for the given optic disc size; a decreased thickness (visibility) of the retinal nerve fiber layer, and a large beta zone of parapapillary atrophy. In a ranking of quantitative optic disc parameters, excluding retinal nerve fiver layer assessment, highest diagnostic power for detecting pre-perimetric glaucoma had the vertical cup/disc diameter ratio corrected for its dependence on optic disc size; total neuroretinal rim area, rim/disc area ratio corrected for disc size, and cup/disc area ratio corrected for disc size. Diagnostic power was lower for rim area in the temporal inferior and temporal superior disc sector, cup area corrected for disc size, and horizontal cup/disc diameter ratio corrected for disc size. Less useful were size of zones alpha and beta of parapapillary chorioretinal atrophy. Due to the overlap between a normal group and patients with early glaucoma, the specificity of quantitative optic disc variables is considerably lower than the specificity of qualitative optic disc variables. For detection of glaucoma, particularly of early glaucoma, qualitative optic disc parameters may, therefore, have higher importance than quantitative variables. The latter will be more important for early detection of progression of the disease than for the early detection of glaucoma as such.

REFERENCES

1. Drance SM, Fairclough M, Butler DM, Kottler MS. The importance of disc hemorrhage in the prognosis of chronic open-angle glaucoma. Arch Ophthalmol, 1977;95:226-228.

2. Airaksinen PJ, Mustonen E, Alanku HI. Optic disc haemorrhages precede retinal nerve fibre layer defects in ocular hypertension. Acta Ophthalmol, 1981;59:627-641

3. Caprioli J, Miller JM, Sears M. Quantitative evaluation of the optic nerve head in patients with unilateral visual field loss from primary open-angle glaucoma. Ophthalmology, 1987; 94: 1484-1487.

4. Sommer A, Katz J, Quigley HA, et al. Clinically detectable nerve fiber atrophy precedes the onset of glaucomatous field loss. Arch Ophthalmol, 1991; 109: 77-83.

5. Quigley HA, Enger C, Katz J, Sommer A, Scott R, Gilbert D. Risk factors for the development of glaucomatous visual field loss in ocular hypertension. Arch Ophthalmol, 1994; 112:644-649.

6. Tezel G, Kolker AE, Kass MA, Wax MB, Gordon M, Siegmund KD. Parapapillary chorioretinal atrophy in patients with ocular hypertension. I. An evaluation as a predictive factor for the development of glaucomatous damage. Arch Ophthalmol, 1997; 115:1503-1508.

7. Bathija R, Zangwill L, Berry CC, Sample P, Weinreb R. Detection of early glaucomatous structural damage with confocal scanning laser tomography. J Glaucoma, 1998; 7: 121-127.

8. Jonas JB, Budde WM, Panda-Jonas S. Ophthalmoscopic evaluation of the optic nerve head. Surv Ophthalmol, 1999; 43: 293-320.

9. Jonas JB, Bergua A, Schmitz-Valckenberg P, Papastathopoulos KI, Budde WM. Ranking of optic disc variables for detection of glaucoma damage. Invest Ophthalmol Vis Sci, 2000; 41: 1764-1773.

Question 18

Glaucoma masqueraders

Leonard A. Levin

What are the main neuro-ophthalmological conditions which can simulate glaucoma?

Any disease of the optic nerve can cause visual loss associated with optic atrophy. Fortunately, there are specific features of the visual loss and optic atrophy associated with glaucoma which distinguish it from the vast majority of optic neuropathies. Specifically, glaucoma has nerve fiber bundle defects because the locus of injury is at the optic disk. These defects, e.g. arcuate scotomas, nasal steps, and temporal wedges, are different from the visual field defects seen in more posterior damage to the optic nerve and/or chiasm, which are typically central scotomas and hemianopic field defects.

The optic atrophy of glaucoma is also unusual, in that there is cupping without significant pallor of the remaining neuroretinal rim. Other optic neuropathies typically cause pallor without cupping. In some cases, cupping (with pallor) can occur, and this can be confused with the appearance of glaucoma. The specific causes of nonglaucomatous disk cupping are listed in Table I.

Other red flags that disk cupping is due to an optic neuropathy other than glaucoma are the following:

1) Loss of color vision, particularly in the red-green axis. Early color vision loss is commonly seen in compressive and inflammatory optic neuropathies, but is rarely seen early in the course in glaucomatous optic neuropathy.

2) Visual acuity loss. Many optic neuropathies cause loss of visual acuity early in the course, but this is unusual in glaucomatous optic neuropathy.

3) Completely asymmetric visual field loss and optic atrophy (where the contralateral side is normal) is relatively unusual in glaucoma, and should raise the suspicion of another process causing the optic neuropathy.

When should neuro-imaging be performed?

Any patient with pallor of the remaining neuroretinal rim or visual field loss that respects the vertical meridian or has a central quality should have neuro-imaging. In addition, patients who have some of the red flags listed in the previous section as having a significant possibility of nonglaucomatous optic neuropathy should also have neuro-imaging. The neuro-imaging should be an MRI scan with and without gadolinium, and should include dedicated views of the orbital optic nerves and chiasm. This will usually require coronal views with fat suppression. The neuroradiologist should be instructed to specifically look for a small meningioma within the confines of the optic canal, as well as other, more obvious abnormalities. Meningiomas are not infrequently seen in patients in the same (elderly) age group where the prevalence of glaucoma is high, and thus the necessity for this mode of imaging. If neuro-imaging is negative and the suspicion of nonglaucomatous optic neuropathy is high, referral to a neuro-ophthalmologist or laboratory testing for other etiologies of anterior visual system disease may be required. In some cases repeated neuro-imaging may be necessary if the optic neuropathy worsens despite therapy.

Table I. Non-Glaucomatous Causes of Disk Cupping
1. Temporal arteritis (arteritic anterior ischemic optic neuropathy)
2. Compressive optic neuropathy (tumor, aneurysm, etc.)
3. Methanol intoxication
4. Shock optic neuropathy (hypotensive optic neuropathy)
5. Kjere optic neuropathy (dominant optic atrophy)
6. Any other optic neuropathy coinciding with a cupped disk.

Question 19

What are the ideal characteristics of a drug for the treatment of primary open angle glaucoma?

Kuldev Singh

This question asks us what characteristics make a drug 'effective' for the treatment of primary open angle glaucoma. Historically, effectiveness and efficacy have been considered to be equivalent to IOP lowering. The greater the degree of IOP lowering, the more effective the drug. For a drug used in the treatment of glaucoma to be ideal, however, it must also possess several other characteristics.

The safety of a medication can never be overemphasized. If a drug has systemic side effects that place the patient's overall health at risk, it should not be considered ideal, regardless of the degree of IOP lowering associated with its use. We have had medications in glaucoma that have, in some instances, been associated with life threatening side effects. In addition, there have been drugs that large groups of patients have not been able to take because of previously existing medical conditions. An ideal glaucoma medication should be systemically safe in all patients.

Besides safety, ocular tolerability is a factor that distinguishes ideal from less than perfect drugs. Significant ocular side effects can have numerous consequences for the patient. For example, a patient may be unwilling to take a drug that causes significant miosis or ocular irritation. Poor compliance is one problem with medications that are not well tolerated. Another relates to the ocular health of eyes that are irritated. It has been postulated that the long term use of glaucoma medications may decrease the ultimate success of glaucoma filtration surgery. An ideal glaucoma

91

medication should be well tolerated and not have harmful ocular side effects.

The dosing schedule of a medication also has the potential to effect compliance. While the difference between once a day and twice daily dosing has not been well studied, there are many who believe that compliance significantly decreases when medications have to be dosed three or more times a day. Dosing once every other day or less frequently has the potential to create confusion, especially since there are an odd number of days in a week. The ideal glaucoma medication should be dosed once daily, either in the morning or evening, whichever is more convenient for the patient.

The cost of glaucoma therapy cannot be ignored, especially in the developing world. If a patient cannot afford or obtain the medication, it is certainly not effective. In addition, the medication should be available in its active form. If loss of potency occurs in the transportation or distribution of a medication, it is also not effective. An ideal glaucoma medication should be affordable, available and easy to administer.

While the answer to the question at hand began by emphasizing that IOP lowering was not the only benchmark which should be used to assess glaucoma therapy, there is no question that this is the only proven way to treat glaucoma. In the future, non IOP lowering therapies may be available and characterize the ideal glaucoma medication. Currently, however, all other things being equal, the greater the degree of IOP lowering associated with a drug, the more desirable it is. The ideal drug for the treatment of primary open angle glaucoma should lower IOP to a level just above the threshold for developing hypotony related ocular problems. This level of IOP varies significantly between patients. A drug that is ideal for one patient may not be safe enough for another. Alternatively, a drug that is safe enough for one patient may not lower IOP enough for another. Patients differ with regard to disease severity, rate of disease progression and life expectancy, with each of these factors being important in determining what constitutes an ideal drug for a given patient.

To summarize, the ideal glaucoma medication should lower IOP as much as possible without causing hypotony. Additionally the medication should have no systemic or ocular side effects and be dosed once a day in the morning or evening, whichever is more convenient for the patient. Ideally, the medication should be affordable and available, in its active form, to all patients. The medication should be easy to administer as topical therapy. No such ideal medication exists today and progress in glaucoma therapeutics is generally slow. Nevertheless, we are closer today to ideal therapy than we have been at any time in the past.

REFERENCES

1. Broadway DC, Grierson I, Hitchings RA. Local effects of previous conjunctival incisional surgery and the subsequent outcome of filtration surgery. Am J Ophthalmol. 1998 Jun;125(6):805-18.

2. Fiscella RG, Green A, Patuszynski DH, Wilensky J. Medical therapy cost considerations for glaucoma Am J Ophthalmol. 2003 Jul;136(1):18-25.

3. Kass, MA, Hodapp E, Gordon M, Kolker AE Goldberg I. Part I. Patient Administration of Eyedrops: Interview. Ann Ophthalmol 14:775, 1982.

4. Kass, MA, Hodapp E, Gordon M, Kolker AE Goldberg I. Patient Administration of Eyedrops: Observation. Part II. Ann Ophthalmol 14:889, 1982.

Question 20

What is maximal tolerated medical therapy?

Robert D. Fechtner

Tony Realini

Maximal tolerated medical therapy (MTMT) originally meant the absolute upper limit of medical therapy possible before causing intolerable adverse effects. This was in an era of glaucoma medications all with notable adverse effect profiles. The unfortunate result was that this meant one had to exceed MTMT and experience adverse effects to find that threshold. Then the final intolerable drug was discontinued in the hope that the remaining drugs would still be tolerable. This approach guaranteed an unpleasant experience for the patient, often with little beneficial additional IOP lowering. In our current practice, we have moved away from MTMT and instead speak of "Maximal Medical Therapy." Alternatively, we have referred to this as "Reasonable Medical Therapy." MTMT can be defined simply as the point at which it makes no sense to add more medication.

The addition of new, effective, convenient glaucoma medications in the past few years has greatly expanded medical therapy options for glaucoma patients. A decade ago, only three classes of topical glaucoma medications were available: beta-blockers, parasympathomimetics, and non-selective adrenenergic agonists (epinephrine) compounds. Oral carbonic anhydrase inhibitors were used quite commonly, often as second or third line therapeutic agents despite their myriad adverse effects. Our treatment paradigm had long been a stepped algorithm with a reasonably obvious order of drug addition. There are now more steps in the algorithm, corresponding to new classes of medications. There are more choices of individual agents within each class, and no longer is the order of addition clear-cut.[1]

How do we know which drugs to add or combine? Ideally, we might rely on peer-reviewed literature to select the best adjunctive medications based on their relative value as additives to our preferred first-line agents. Unfortunately, our literature lacks much of the necessary data, either because studies comparing additivities of newer drugs have not been performed, or because many published pre- and post-marketing studies are flawed and of limited value in making clinical management decisions.[2]

Does this mean we should advance treatment to one medication from each class in all patients prior to trying other treatment modalities such as laser trabeculoplasty or glaucoma filtration surgery? Does it mean we should continue adding medications in pursuit of lowest IOP until the patient suffers adverse effects? Obviously not! We are looking for therapeutic benefit while minimizing adverse effects. Maximal medical therapy could be redefined as the maximum combination of drugs likely to provide clinically significant additive IOP-lowering effect.

It is well worth recognizing that there are differing situations with which we are faced that result in the decision to treat with more than one drug. When a patient is newly diagnosed, we set a target IOP based on patient factors and our judgment. If initial monotherapy is ineffective, we should switch to a drug in a different class. However, if an effective drug does not achieve the target, or if the target is very low, we may need to use additional medications. Similarly, when a patient is at target, but has progression of glaucoma, we adjust the target downward and advance therapy.

While we readily add a second drug when the first is not providing the desired effect, we must recognize that glaucoma medications in different classes that are effective as monotherapy are not always significantly additive. We have, in recent years, depended on the one-eye trial to demonstrate the efficacy of the additive therapy.

As a rule, the magnitude of IOP lowering (either in mm Hg or percentage) is greatest with the first agent. Typically, we expect 20-30% reduction in IOP from an effective drug as monotherapy with only 10-15% from the next drug added. There are reasons for this. The IOP lowering effect of most glaucoma medications is pressure dependent; the higher the IOP, the greater the IOP lowering effect. Thus it is not surprising that we see One would thus expect diminishing returns when sequentially adding medications on top of others that have already lowered IOP significantly. This has been demonstrated in several studies.

In recent years the non-selective beta-adrenergic antagonists were the most common choice for initial monotherapy. Many ophthalmologists now favor a prostaglandin analog as monotherapy. Other drugs that are popular as adjuncts are topical carbonic anhydrase inhibitors and alpha-2 adrenergic agonists. We cannot provide much guidance as to which combinations are likely the most effective as evidence is lacking. We do note that the availability of fixed-combination drugs can simplify dosing regimens.

Maximal or reasonable medical therapy must be individualized for each patient. We do this by setting a target pressure for each patient (and often for each eye).[3] We then select primary therapy based on safety, efficacy, ease of administration, and cost. From the medical history we learn of drug contraindications, concurrent health issues, conflicting medication use, or allergies. A patient's age and health status help us to estimate the length of therapeutic effect required. A social history helps us rate the consequences of side effects of a particular eyedrop. And of course, from our examinations and ancillary testing, we learn the severity and rate of progression of their disease. All this information is integrated to formulate a goal target-IOP range within which we expect no further progression, excepting that from aging itself. Since target-IOP ranges are just educated guesses, we remain obligated to continue monitoring for progression even if the target is reached, and continually adjust therapy and revise the IOP goal, usually down, as necessary.

For those with insufficient IOP control on medical therapy, the question remains, when does one stop adding medications and consider surgical options? Some ophthalmologists simply do not like to do glaucoma surgery and will continue adding drugs in the absence of a clinically meaningful drop in IOP. We urge clinicians to discontinue drugs that are not effective. Proceeding to filtration surgery after combining three or perhaps four classes of medications certainly seems a conservative approach. But is it a rational approach? Most ophthalmologists prescribe at least two glaucoma medications prior to considering surgical intervention. After the second, and certainly after the third drug is prescribed, it is difficult to make a good case for continuing to add medications.[4]

How much is enough? Most glaucoma patients should be treated with the one or two agents that best lower IOP. The individual therapeutic trial remains crucial to guide therapy; especially when there is little data to help in the selection. If you are thinking of adding a third agent, consider laser trabeculoplasty, or incisional surgery. Most patients will not need to go beyond a combination product, plus one additional agent; two bottles and three or four drops per day is enough. Three or four bottles are usually too much of a good thing.

REFERENCES

1. Realini T, Fechtner RD. 56,000 ways to treat glaucoma. Ophthalmology, 2002; 109(11): 1955-6.

2. Camras CB, Minckler D. Does that drug work? Pitfalls in studies on the efficacy and safety of glaucoma medications. [editorial] Am J Ophthalmol, 2000;129(1):87-89.

3. Realini T, Fechtner RD. Target intraocular pressure in glaucoma management. Ophthalmology Clinics of North America, 2000; 13(3):407-15.

4. Fechtner RD, Singh K. Maximal glaucoma therapy. Journal of Glaucoma, 2001; 10:S73-S75.

Question 21

What is the practical importance of blood flow evaluation in glaucoma?

Makoto Araie

To discuss this issue, it must be first stated that glaucoma referred in this chapter is limited to open angle glaucoma (OAG) including classical primary open angle glaucoma and normal-tension glaucoma (NTG). There are several risk factors for OAG; Intraocular pressure (IOP) that is probably the most important risk factor, age, race, myopia, genetic disposition or presence of family history of OAG, and blood flow-related risk factor(s).[1] Among them, only the IOP and blood flow related risk factor are those which can be modified by treatment.

Relationship exists between low systemic blood pressure, especially low ocular perfusion pressure and OAG,[2] between migrane and vasospastic syndrome and OAG on the normal-tension side. Noctural hypotension is also linked to progression of OAG.[3] Relationship between progression or extent of damage of OAG and presence of optic disc hemorrhage, peripapillary atrophy or choroidal sclerosis as presumed local blood flow-related risk factors has been reported, and reduced ocular or retrobulbar blood flow has been also suggested in many of OAG patients.[4] Glaucomatous damage in the optic nerve head (ONH) or retinal nerve fiber layer should lead to secondary blood flow-related changes, but it must be noted that there is a report suggesting that local blood flow-related change may precede the visual field damage in OAG.[5] These clinical facts suggest that systemic or local blood flow evaluation in OAG patients may be helpful to know whether the patient is at more risk of future progression.

It is possible to modify some of the blood flow-related risk factors. Ocular perfusion pressure can be increased by lowering IOP by medical or surgical therapy, though it is difficult for eye doctors to modify systemic blood pressure. It is also possible to improve blood flow in ocular tissues including ONH in human eyes by drugs of which clinical long-term safety have been established in other fields of medicine.[6] Several preliminary clinical studies suggested that such drugs may lead to improvement of visual field performance during the study-period at least in a part of patients.[7,8] Needless to say that these preliminary findings need validation by future randomized clinical trials, but the possibility that progression of OAG is retarded by improving blood flow irrespective of IOP lowering can not be excluded.

Then, how can we non-invasively evaluate ocular blood flow in our OAG patients? Color Doppler imaging (CDI) allows us to measure the blood flow velocity in the central retinal artery or short posterior ciliary arteries nourishing posterior choroid and prelaminar and laminar portions of the ONH. Laser Doppler velocimetry (LDV) measures the blood flow velocity and blood flow rate through major retinal vessels. (Scanning) laser Doppler flowmetry (LDF) and laser speckle method allow us to estimate blood flow in the choroid and ONH at least to a depth of its prelaminar portion in arbitrary units. On the other hand, pulsatile ocular blood flow measurements only give a blood flow parameter mainly representing whole choroidal blood flow, and angiographic methods which need intravenous injection of dyes are not sufficiently safe. Both CDI and LDV give absolute values of blood flow parameters, which makes inter-individual or ye comparison possible. However, blood flow in the ONH where glaucomatous damage takes place can be directly evaluated by these methods. On the other hand, both LDF and laser speckle method give only relative (not absolute) values of blood blow, which makes these methods suited for intra-individual or ye comparison, but not for inter-individual or ye comparison.

Now, we must consider what practical (non-academic) importance of blood flow evaluation with CDI or sophisticated laser-using methods in our OAG patients is. At present time of investigation, causal relationship between reduced perfusion and glaucomatous optic neuropathy is not established, nor effects of blood flow improving therapy on the prognosis of OAG. Whatever the results of blood flow measurement are, eyes or patients where active modification of systemic circulation is justified seem rather limited to those with sufficiently lowered IOP, but showing rapid progression or suffering impending loss of the central vision.

There are reports indicating that in monkey or rabbit eyes topically instilled drugs modify the ONH or retinal blood flow by locally penetrating to the posterior segments of the eye at pharmacologically active levels.[9,10] If this is also the case in human eyes, and topically instilled drugs which can modify the ONH or retinal blood flow by their local effects to clinically significant levels become available, then blood flow evaluation in OAG patients will become practically more important.

REFERENCES

1. Shields MB. Textbook of Glaucoma (4th ed.). Baltimore: Williams & Wilkins, 1997.

2. Tielsch JM, Katz J, Sommer A, Quigley HA, Javitt JC. Hypertension, perfusion pressure, and primary open angle glaucoma. A population-based assessment. Arch Ophthalmol, 1995;113:216-221

3. Hayreh SS, Zimmerman MB, Podhajsky P, Alward WLM. Nocturnal arterial hypotension and its role in optic nerve head and ocular ischemic disorder. Am J Ophthalmol, 1994;117:603-624

4. Flammer J. The vascular concept of glaucoma. Surv Ophthalmol, 1994;38:3-6

5. Nicolera MT, Drance SM, Rankin SJA, Buckley AR, Walman BE. Color Dopper imaging in patients with asymmetric glaucoma and unilateral visual field loss. Am J Ophthalmol, 1996;121:502-510

6. Tomita K, Araie M, Tamaki Y, Nagahara M, Sugiyama T. Effects of nilvadipine, a calcium antagonist, on rabbit ocular circulation and optic never head circulation in normal tension glaucoma subjects. Investigative Ophthalmology & Visual Science, 40: 1144-1151,1999

7. Netland PA, Chaturvedi N, Dreyer EB. Calcium-channel blockers in the management of low-tension and open-angle glaucoma. Am J Ophthalmol, 1993;115:608-613.

8. Sawada A, Kitazawa Y, Yamamoto T, Okabe I, Ichien K. Prevention of visual field defect progression with brovincamine in eyes with normal-tension glaucoma. Ophthalmology, 1996;103:283-288

9. Mizuno K, Koide T, Saito N, Fujii M, Nagahara M, Tomidokoro A, Tamaki Y, Araie M. Topical nipradilol: effects on optic nerve head circulation in humans and periocular distribution in monkeys. Investigative Ophthalmology & Visual Science, 2002;43:3243-3250

10. Ishii K, Matsuo H, Fukaya Y, Tanaka S, Sakai H, Waki M, Araie M. Iganidipine, A New Water-Soluble Ca2+ Antagonist. Ocular and Periocular Penetration after Instillation. Investigative Ophthalmology & Visual Science, 2003;44:1169-1177

Question 22

Is a glaucoma vaccination feasible? (Towards development of a vaccination for glaucoma)

Michal Schwartz

Introduction

During the past decade scientists and clinicians began to accept that glaucoma should not be viewed as a distinct syndrome with its own peculiar features, but as part of the large group of neurodegenerative disorders of the central nervous system (CNS) that are characterized by a primary loss of neurons caused by one or more risk factors, and an ongoing process of secondary degeneration triggered as a result of the primary loss (Schwartz et al., 1996; Schwartz and Yoles, 2000a, b; Schwartz and Kipnis, 2002). This view of glaucoma has led to major changes in the nature of glaucoma research, the way in which clinicians perceive the disease, and the approach to therapy (Kaufman et al., 1999; Quigley, 1999; Mittag et al., 2000; Weinreb, 2001). The emphasis, instead of being mainly on the primary risk factors and their effect on the optic neurons, has shifted towards the hostility created by the primary insult, with consequent progression of secondary degeneration even if that particular etiological factor is adequately neutralized. Most of the current research effort is therefore aimed at identifying the compounds and factors responsible for mediating the self-perpetuating degeneration and seeking ways to circumvent or block them.

In the course of these studies it has become clear that some of the compounds identified in the pathogenesis of glaucoma are already known to be active in other neurodegenerative diseases. Research findings in connection with other neurodegenerative conditions have therefore influenced the direction of research on glaucoma. Our own studies of acute and chronic injuries of the rodent optic nerve led us to discover that a key role in the ability of the optic nerve and the retina to withstand injurious conditions is played by the immune system.

T cells directed to self-antigens residing in the site of injury mediate the ability to fight off degeneration

Our first observations that the immune system (in the form of T cells directed to certain self-antigens) can protect injured neurons from death came from studies in rodents showing that passive transfer of T cells specific to myelin basic protein (MBP) reduces the loss of retinal ganglion cells after a traumatic injury. We found that these T cells are also effective when directed to either cryptic or pathogenic epitopes of MBP, as well as to other myelin antigens or their epitopes. These findings raised a number of critical questions (Moalem et al., 1999b; Moalem et al., 1999a; Schwartz et al., 1999; Hauben et al., 2000; Moalem et al., 2000; Yoles et al., 2001). For example, are myelin antigens capable of protecting the visual system from any type of acute or chronic insult? Is the observed neuroprotective activity of immune cells merely an anecdotal finding reflecting our experimental conditions, or does it point to the critical participation of the immune system in fighting off injurious conditions in the visual system and in the CNS in general? If the latter, can this participation be translated into a neuroprotective therapy?

In a series of experiments carried out over the last few years we have learned, firstly, that the protective effect of vaccination with myelin-associated antigens is restricted to injuries of the white matter, i.e., to myelinated axons (Schori et al., 2001; Mizrahi et al., 2002). If the insult is to the retina, which contains no myelin, myelin antigens have no effect. Secondly, we observed that the injury-induced response of T cells reactive to specific self-antigens residing in the site of stress (eye or brain) is a spontaneous physiological response. This response might be sufficient to overcome the threat (without the individual's even being aware that protection was needed and provided), or insufficient (with consequent progression of degeneration), or defective (and therefore contributing to the neuronal loss). We then sought to identify the phenotype of the beneficial autoimmune T cells and to understand what determines the balance between a beneficial (neuroprotective) outcome of the T cell-mediated response to a CNS injury and a destructive effect causing autoimmune disease. We also examined ways of translating the beneficial response into a therapy for glaucoma. Some critical aspects had to be addressed along the way: (1) We verified that the loss of retinal ganglion cells in a rat model of high intraocular pressure, simulating some types of glaucoma, is T cell-dependent. (2) We attempted to determine whether the specific self-antigens that are harnessed by the protective autoimmune T cells in our rat model of chronic glaucoma, and which can be boosted for therapeutic purposes, reside in the retina or the optic nerve. (3) We searched for an antigen that would be able to safely boost the physiological response without causing an autoimmune disease.

Using our rat model of chronic glaucoma, we showed that a protective response could be obtained only with an antigen residing in the retina, suggesting that at least in this model the site of self-perpetuating degeneration, and therefore the site in need of protection, is not the optic nerve but the retina.

The mechanism underlying T cell-dependent neuroprotection without autoimmune disease

Having established that the body recruit autoimmune T cells to help fight off degenerative conditions, we attempted to find out what determines the differences between protective and destructive autoimmunity. We discovered that both protective and destructive autoimmunity can potentially be mediated by T cells of identical phenotype and specificity, or in other words, by the same helper T cells (Th1).

Our results suggest that a sub-population of naturally occurring regulatory T cells (CD4+CD25+) is responsible for balancing the need for autoimmunity with the risk of autoimmune disease. In situations where the need for autoimmune protection is not fully met, the regulation is shifted so as to increase the number of autoimmune T cells potentially available for action. Until recently, suppression of autoimmune disease was attributed to the suppressive effect of this sub-population of regulatory T cells on autoimmune T cells. Our results suggest, however, that the function of the regulatory T cells is to maintain a balance that allows protection (i.e., beneficial autoimmunity) but not autoimmune disease (i.e., destructive autoimmunity) to be expressed (Kipnis et al., 2002; Kipnis et al., 2004).

Given that self-perpetuating degeneration is a multi-parameter process invoking the participation of numerous factors, it seems reasonable to assume that the multidimensional approach provided by an immune cell-based therapy will be superior to any drug treatment capable of addressing only one or very few aspects of the risk factors involved (Schori et al., 2001b; Schori et al., 2001a; Schori et al., 2002b; Schori et al., 2002a).

When designing immune intervention to boost neuroprotection, the risk of autoimmune disease can be avoided by the use of an antigen comprising a nonpathogenic sequence derived from a relevant self-protein that may itself be pathogenic. Suitable antigens might be crytic epitopes or altered peptides (Moalem et al., 1999b; Fisher et al., 2001; Hauben et al., 2001; Mizrahi et al., 2002). Also promising is a synthetic antigen such as Cop-1, which is weakly cross-reactive with a wide range of self-antigens residing in the eye or in the nerve, and was found experimentally by our group to be effective in boosting neuroprotection in rodents suffering from glaucoma Cop-1, administered on a daily basis, is an approved drug for multiple sclerosis, and can thus be considered safe for human consumption, i.e. it does not induce an autoimmune disease (Kipnis et al., 2000; Schori et al., 2001b; Bakalash et al., 2002). Therefore, development of an appropriate regimen for therapy with Cop-1 against glaucoma can be started immediately. Other suitable antigens besides Cop-1 are also being sought.

REFERENCES

1. Bakalash S, Kipnis J, Yoles E, Schwartz M (2002) Resistance of retinal ganglion cells to an increase in intraocular pressure is immune-dependent. Invest Ophthalmol Vis Sci 43:2648-2653.

2. Fisher J, Levkovitch-Verbin H, Schori H, Yoles E, Butovsky O, Kaye JF, Ben-Nun A, Schwartz M (2001) Vaccination for neuroprotection in the mouse optic nerve: implications for optic neuropathies. J Neurosci 21:136-142.

3. Hauben E, Agranov E, Gothilf A, Nevo U, Cohen A, Smirnov I, Steinman L, Schwartz M (2001) Posttraumatic therapeutic vaccination with modified myelin self-antigen prevents complete paralysis while avoiding autoimmune disease. J Clin Invest 108:591-599.

4. Hauben E, Butovsky O, Nevo U, Yoles E, Moalem G, Agranov E, Mor F, Leibowitz-Amit R, Pevsner E, Akselrod S, Neeman M, Cohen IR, Schwartz M (2000) Passive or active

immunization with myelin basic protein promotes recovery from spinal cord contusion. J Neurosci 20:6421-6430.

5. Kaufman PL, Gabelt BT, Cynader M (1999) Introductory comments on neuroprotection. Surv Ophthalmol 43 Suppl 1:S89-90.

6. Kipnis, J, Cardon M, Avidan H, Lewitus GM, Mordechay S, Rolls A, Shani Y, Schwartz M (2004) Dopamine, through the extracellular signal-regulated kinase pathway, downregulates CD4+CD25+ regulatory T-cell activity: implications for neurodegeneration. J Neurosci 24:6133-6143.

7. Kipnis J, Mizrahi T, Hauben E, Shaked I, Shevach E, Schwartz M (2002) Neuroprotective autoimmunity: Naturally occurring CD4+CD25+ regulatory T cells suppress the ability to withstand injury to the central nervous system. Proc Natl Acad Sci USA 99:15620-15625.

8. Kipnis J, Yoles E, Porat Z, Cohen A, Mor F, Sela M, Cohen IR, Schwartz M (2000) T cell immunity to copolymer 1 confers neuroprotection on the damaged optic nerve: possible therapy for optic neuropathies. Proc Natl Acad Sci U S A 97:7446-7451.

9. Mittag TW, Danias J, Pohorenec G, Yuan HM, Burakgazi E, Chalmers-Redman R, Podos SM, Tatton WG (2000) Retinal damage after 3 to 4 months of elevated intraocular pressure in a rat glaucoma model. Invest Ophthalmol Vis Sci 41:3451-3459.

10. Mizrahi T, Hauben E, Schwartz M (2002) The tissue-specific self-pathogen is the protective self-antigen: The case of uveitis. J Immunol 169:5971-5977.

11. Moalem G, Monsonego A, Shani Y, Cohen IR, Schwartz M (1999a) Differential T cell response in central and peripheral nerve injury: connection with immune privilege. Faseb J 13:1207-1217.

12. Moalem G, Leibowitz-Amit R, Yoles E, Mor F, Cohen IR, Schwartz M (1999b) Autoimmune T cells protect neurons from secondary degeneration after central nervous system axotomy. Nat Med 5:49-55.

13. Moalem G, Gdalyahu A, Shani Y, Otten U, Lazarovici P, Cohen IR, Schwartz M (2000) Production of neurotrophins by activated T cells: implications for neuroprotective autoimmunity. J Autoimmun 15:331-345.

14. Quigley HA (1999) Neuronal death in glaucoma. Prog Retin Eye Res 18:39-57.

15. Schori H, Yoles E, Schwartz M (2001a) T-cell-based immunity counteracts the potential toxicity of glutamate in the central nervous system. J Neuroimmunol 119:199-204.

16. Schori H, Yoles E, Wheeler LA, Schwartz M (2002a) Immune related mechanisms participating in resistance and susceptibility to glutamate toxicity. Eur J Neurosci 16:557-564.

17. Schori H, Lantner F, Shachar I, Schwartz M (2002b) Severe immunodeficiency has opposite effects on neuronal survival in glutamate-susceptible and -resistant mice: Adverse effect of B cells. J Immunol 169:2861-2865.

18. Schori H, Kipnis J, Yoles E, WoldeMussie E, Ruiz G, Wheeler LA, Schwartz M (2001b) Vaccination for protection of retinal ganglion cells against death from glutamate cytotoxicity and ocular hypertension: implications for glaucoma. Proc Natl Acad Sci U S A 98:3398-3403.

19. Schwartz M, Yoles E (2000a) Self-destructive and self-protective processes in the damaged optic nerve: implications for glaucoma. Invest Ophthalmol Vis Sci 41:349-351.

20. Schwartz M, Yoles E (2000b) Neuroprotection: a new treatment modality for glaucoma? Curr Opin Ophthalmol 11:107-111.

21. Schwartz M, Kipnis J (2002) Prospects for therapeutic vaccination with glatiramer acetate for neurodegenerative diseases such as Alzheimer's disease. Drug Dev Res 56:143-149.

22. Schwartz M, Belkin M, Yoles E, Solomon A (1996) Potential treatment modalities for glaucomatous neuropathy: neuroprotection and neuroregeneration. J Glaucoma 5:427-432.

23. Schwartz M, Moalem G, Leibowitz-Amit R, Cohen IR (1999) Innate and adaptive immune responses can be beneficial for CNS repair. Trends Neurosci 22:295-299.

24. Weinreb RN (2001) Neuroprotection—possibilities in perspective. Surv Ophthalmol 45 Suppl 3:S241-242.

25. Yoles E, Hauben E, Palgi O, Agranov E, Gothilf A, Cohen A, Kuchroo V, Cohen IR, Weiner H, Schwartz M (2001) Protective autoimmunity is a physiological response to CNS trauma. J Neurosci 21:3740-3748.

Question 23

When should we treat ocular hypertensives?

K. Schwartz

Richard K. Parrish

The Ocular Hypertension Treatment Study (OHTS) findings, published in June 2002, have resulted in a major paradigm shift for decision making in the treatment of ocular hypertension.[1,2] Prior to OHTS, ocular hypertension treatment was based on individual physician experience more than sound science. Although the relationship between elevated intraocular pressure (IOP) and the development of primary open angle glaucoma (POAG) had been previously reported, no definitive or widely accepted guidelines existed.[3,4] Several studies reported conflicting results on the question of whether IOP lowering prevented or delayed the development of POAG.[5-13] All studies demonstrated that a small percentage of untreated ocular hypertensive patients developed glaucoma; however, no predictive risk factors were identified. The OHTS confirmed that 9.5% of untreated ocular hypertensives developed either optic nerve damage or visual field loss after 5 years, compared with 4.4% of patients who had been treated with drops to reduce IOP by 20%.

Understanding which ocular hypertensive patients are at highest risk to develop damage helps the ophthalmologist to target treatment to those who would be most likely to benefit. The question of "When should we treat ocular hypertensives?" more relevantly stated becomes "Which ocular hypertensive patients should be treated?".

The OHTS reported baseline demographic and clinical examination characteristics that can be used to estimate a risk profile for individual patients. Older age, larger vertical and horizontal cup-disc ratio, pattern standard deviation, and higher IOP at baseline, are risk factors for the development of POAG. Central corneal thickness was a powerful predictor for future damage: the thinner the central cornea the higher the risk. The OHTS findings can be used to categorize patients in to lower and higher risk groups. The lower risk group characteristics include patients with central corneal thickness >588, small vertical cup - disc ratio (less than 0.2), and IOP less than 24 mm Hg. Patients with these baseline characteristics had approximately a 2% chance of developing POAG over the first 5 years of the study. The higher risk group includes patients with central corneal thickness <555 microns, baseline IOP >27.75 mm Hg, and cup - disc ratio 0.5 or greater.

In making the decision of when to treat ocular hypertension, we must compare the risk and costs of treatment versus the benefits of preventing POAG. Although older patients are more likely to develop POAG, the shorter life expectancy, importance of general health issues, and possible systemic side effects of topical medications must be considered. Lundberg reported that 34% of 41 ocular hypertensive patients who were followed prospectively for 20 years developed POAG. [12] The longer the exposure to elevated IOP, the higher the rate of conversion. The OHTS has followed all patients for a minimum of approximately 6 years. Based on the initial findings, *all* patients are being treated in OHTS II to determine if the delay in lowering IOP resulted in an ongoing higher risk of developing POAG.

The OHTS demonstrated that IOP lowering by 20% from baseline levels delayed or prevented the development of POAG. Although the number need to treat was approximately 20, (100/5.1), the actual benefits are much higher for those with the high risk factors. The OHTS does not address the question if greater IOP reduction, such as 25 or 30%, would have resulted in a greater protection.

Based on these findings we recommend the measurement of central corneal thickness in all ocular hypertensive patients and the initiation of IOP lowering in the group of patients who are older, with IOP >28 mm Hg, cup-disc ratio 0.5 or greater, and central corneal thickness >555 microns.

REFERENCES

1. Kass MA, Heuer DK, Higginbotham EJ, et al. The Ocular Hypertension Treatment Study: a randomized trial determines that topical ocular hypotensigve medication de-

lays or prevents the onset of primary open-angle glaucoma. Arch Ophthalmol. 2002;1220:701-713.

2. Gordon MO, Beiser JA, Brandt JD, et al. Ocular Hypertension Treatment Study. Baseline Factors that Predict the Onset of Primary Open-Angle Glaucoma. Arch Ophthalmol. 2002;120:714-720.

3. Hollows FC, Graham PA. Intraocular pressure, glaucoma and glaucoma suspects in a defined population. Br J Ophthalmol. 1966;50:570-586

4. Anderson DR. Glaucoma: the damage caused by pressure. XLVI Edward Jackson Memorial Lecture. Am J Ophthalmology 1989;108:485-95.

5. Armaly MF. Ocular pressure and visual fields: a ten-year follow up study. Arch Ophthalmol. 1969;81:25-40.

6. Norskov K. Routine tonometry in ophthalmic practice. Five year follow-up. Acta Ophthalmol. 1970;48:873-95.

7. Perkins ES. The Bedford Glaucoma Survey I. Long-tern follow up of borderline cases. Brit J Ophthalmol. 1973:57:179-185.

8. Wilensky JT, Podos SM, Becker B. Prognostic indicators in ocular hypertension. Acta Ophthalmol. 1974;91:200-202.

9. Bengtsson B. The prevalence of glaucoma. Br J Ophthalmol. 1981;65:46-49.

10. Kitazawa Y. Prophylactic therapy of ocular hypertension: a prospective study. Trans Ophthalmol Soc NZ 1981;33:30-2.

11. Hovding G, Aasved H. Prognostic factors in the development of manifest open angle glaucoma. Acta Ophthalmol. 1986;64:601-608.

12. Lundberg L, Wettrell K, Linner E. Ocular hypertension. A prospective twenty-year follow-up study. Acta Ophthalmologica. 1987;65:705-708.

13. Heijl A, Bengtsson B. Long term effects of timolol therapy in ocular hypertension: a double-masked, randomized trial. Graefes Arch Clin Exp Ophthalmol. 2000;238:877-883.

Question 24

What is the practical importance of pachymetry in the clinical evaluation of glaucoma?

James D. Brandt

Goldmann applanation tonometry (GAT) has been regarded for almost a half century as the "gold standard' of IOP measurement. Goldmann and Schmidt acknowledged that their design assumptions were based on a central corneal thickness (CCT) of 500 µm and that the accuracy of their device would vary if CCT deviated from this value.[1] Given the paucity of published data at the time, 500 µm seemed a reasonable assumption for the 'average' patient. We now know CCT varies greatly among the general population, to a degree that impacts the accuracy of GAT in daily practice.

In 1975, Ehlers cannulated 29 otherwise normal eyes undergoing cataract surgery and correlated corneal thickness with errors in GAT.[2] He found that GAT most accurately reflected 'true' intracameral IOP when CCT was 520 µm, and that deviations from this value resulted in an over- or under-estimation of IOP by as much as 7 mmHg per 100 µm. Numerous investigators have since demonstrated that CCT varies far more among otherwise normal individuals than Goldmann and Schmidt ever dreamed;[3-6] differences in CCT are seen among different racial and ethnic groups,[7,8] can lead to mis-classification of patients with normal tension glaucoma[9-11] and ocular hypertension.[9,12-14] The importance of CCT in the management of glaucoma patients, particularly those with ocular hypertension, was recently driven home by findings from the Ocular Hypertension Treatment Study (OHTS).[15-17]

In the OHTS, patients were recruited who had *untreated* GAT measurements in one eye between 24 and 32 mmHg on two separate

113

occasions (the other had to be between 21 and 32 mmHg), with no secondary cause of elevated IOP. The patients all had normal visual fields and optic nerves. CCT was measured approximately two years after enrollment was completed. Among the OHTS participants, 25% had CCT values above 600 μm.[15] If one uses Ehler's correction of 7 mmHg/100 μM deviation from the nominal value of 520 μM, then as many as 50% of OHTS subjects had 'corrected' IOP values upon entry below 21 mmHg. In a multivariate model of baseline characteristics predictive of which subjects would develop glaucoma, CCT proved to be the most potent.[17]

The OHTS results demonstrate that many patients are being mis-classified in terms of glaucoma risk on the basis of erroneous IOP estimates by GAT. Clearly, many individuals with elevated GAT measurements but no other findings suggestive of glaucoma probably have normal 'true' IOPs and do not need treatment or even increased glaucoma surveillance. What about patients with established glaucoma? Can CCT provide the clinician with data to help refine target pressures?

Weizer and co-workers recently performed a retrospective review of all newly-referred glaucoma patients over several years.[18] In both univariate and multivariate analyses, CCT had a stronger (inverse) relationship to the degree of glaucoma damage than anything else, including IOP! The implication of this finding is that patients with thin corneas have higher IOPs than are appreciated by the clinicians caring for them – in a patient with advanced disease and a CCT of 480 μm, perhaps the clinician should not consider a GAT measurement of 16 mmHg as acceptable.

The question of whether a validated 'correction algorithm' exists is, in my opinion, not particularly important in daily practice. The clinician should be cautious in extrapolating Ehlers' findings to general clinical practice. His study was based on a small number of eyes (29) that included a relatively narrow range of CCTs (450 to 590 μm).[2] The interested reader is referred to a detailed exploration of the mechanical characteristics of the cornea and the role of CCT in GAT error by Orssengo and Pye[19] in which a mathematical and engineering model closely approximates Ehlers' and other published cannulation data. Based on this and the OHTS findings it is my opinion that Ehlers' estimate is probably close to the magnitude of error that occurs in real life. If there is one thing I've learned over the past few years of performing pachymetry on most of my patients is that one can take far better care of patients simply by categorizing corneas as 'thin, average or thick', just as it is important to recognize that optic discs come in 'small, medium and large', allowing the clinician to interpret disc configurations accordingly. Measuring CCT leads to the discontinuation of therapy in many over-treated ocular hypertensives and escalation of therapy in patients with thin corneas in whom control is clearly inadequate. Ultimately, incorporating the measurement of CCT into the glaucoma exam allows the astute clinician to better target and titrate the treatment of glaucoma.

REFERENCES

1. Goldmann H, Schmidt T. Über applanationstonometrie. Ophthalmologica, 1957; 134: 221-242.

2. Ehlers N, Bramsen T, Sperling S. Applanation tonometry and central corneal thickness. Acta Ophthalmol (Copenh), 1975;53:34-43.

3. Alsbirk PH. Corneal thickness. I. Age variation, sex difference and oculometric correlations. Acta Ophthalmol (Copenh), 1978;56:95-104.

4. Wolfs RC, Klaver CC, Vingerling JR, Grobbee DE, Hofman A, de Jong PT. Distribution of central corneal thickness and its association with intraocular pressure: The Rotterdam Study. Am J Ophthalmol, 1997;123:767-72.

5. Whitacre MM, Stein RA, Hassanein K. The effect of corneal thickness on applanation tonometry. American Journal of Ophthalmology, 1993;115:592-6.

6. Stodtmeister R. Applanation tonometry and correction according to corneal thickness. Acta Ophthalmol Scand, 1998;76:319-24.

7. Foster PJ, Baasanhu J, Alsbirk PH, Munkhbayar D, Uranchimeg D, Johnson GJ. Central corneal thickness and intraocular pressure in a Mongolian population. Ophthalmology, 1998;105:969-73.

8. La Rosa FA, Gross RL, Orengo-Nania S. Central corneal thickness of Caucasians and African Americans in glaucomatous and nonglaucomatous populations. Archives of Ophthalmology, 2001;119:23-7.

9. Copt RP, Thomas R, Mermoud A. Corneal thickness in ocular hypertension, primary open-angle glaucoma, and normal tension glaucoma [see comments]. Arch Ophthalmol, 1999;117:14-6.

10. Ehlers N, Hansen FK. Central corneal thickness in low-tension glaucoma. Acta Ophthalmol (Copenh), 1974;52:740-6.

11. Emara BY, Tingey DP, Probst LE, Motolko MA. Central corneal thickness in low-tension glaucoma. Canadian Journal of Ophthalmology, 1999;34:319-24.

12. Argus WA. Ocular hypertension and central corneal thickness. Ophthalmology, 1995; 102:1810-2.

13. Bron AM, Creuzot-Garcher C, Goudeau-Boutillon S, d'Athis P. Falsely elevated intraocular pressure due to increased central corneal thickness. Graefes Arch Clin Exp Ophthalmol, 1999;237:220-4.

14. Herndon LW, Choudhri SA, Cox T, Damji KF, Shields MB, Allingham RR. Central corneal thickness in normal, glaucomatous, and ocular hypertensive eyes [see comments]. Arch Ophthalmol, 1997;115:1137-41.

15. Brandt JD, Beiser JA, Kass MA, Gordon MO. Central Corneal Thickness in the Ocular Hypertension Treatment Study (OHTS). Ophthalmology, 2001;108:1779-1788.

16. Kass MA, Heuer DK, Higginbotham EJ, et al. The Ocular Hypertension Treatment Study: A Randomized Trial Determines That Topical Ocular Hypotensive Medication Delays or Prevents the Onset of Primary Open-Angle Glaucoma. Arch Ophthalmol, 2002;120:701-713.

17. Gordon MO, Beiser JA, Brandt JD, et al. The Ocular Hypertension Treatment Study: Baseline Factors That Predict the Onset of Primary Open-Angle Glaucoma. Arch Ophthalmol, 2002;120:714-720.

18. Weizer J, Stinnett S, Herndon LW. Central corneal thickness as a risk factor for advanced glaucoma damage. Arch Ophthalmol, 2003:in press.

19. Orssengo GJ, Pye DC. Determination of the true intraocular pressure and modulus of elasticity of the human cornea in vivo. Bull Mathematical Biol, 1999;61:551-572.

Are myopic eyes more susceptible to glaucomatous damage?

Claude F. Burgoyne

Two questions should frame the discussion regarding myopia and glaucoma. First, do myopic eyes have an increased prevalence of elevated eye pressure and, second, is the myopic optic nerve head more susceptible to IOP-related damage at all levels of IOP?

Do myopic eyes have an increased prevalence of elevated IOP?

A series of studies have reported higher IOP levels in myopic eyes or increased risk of ocular hypertension in myopic eyes.[1] Within the 3654 participants of the Blue Mountains Eye Study, Mitchell and co-authors[2] reported an increased risk for ocular hypertension in the low (greater than or equal to -1D to less than -3D) (but not the moderate to high) myopic group. However, Daubs and Crick,[3] in a case-control study of nearly 1000 eyes, did not find a relationship between IOP and low or high myopia, and Bengtsson[4] found that the relationship became insignificant when he controlled for additional variables such as blood pressure, sex, season and time of day.

Are myopic eyes more susceptible to glaucomatous damage at all levels of IOP?

From an engineering standpoint, there are several reasons why the myopic optic nerve head should be more susceptible to a given level of IOP. First, the myopic scleral canal may be unusually large, abnormally shaped, and/or tilted, leading to elevated levels of IOP-related stress for a given level of

IOP.[5] Second, the myopic lamina[6] and peripapillary sclera[5] may be unusually thin, leading to higher IOP-related scleral wall stress and deformation. Third, the extracellular matrix of myopic sclera may be abnormally weak, causing larger scleral deformations for a given level of IOP. Fourth, the size of the axially myopic eye (separate from the thinning of the sclera) should increase IOP-related scleral stress for a given level of IOP.[5]

The following clinical relationships, if present, would support the notion that an axially myopic eye is more susceptible to both normal and elevated levels of IOP: 1) an increased prevalence of normal pressure glaucoma in myopes, 2) an increased risk for ocular hypertensive myopes to convert to glaucomatous damage, and 3) an increased rate of glaucomatous progression in myopic COAG patients.

Two studies have found an increased risk for the presence of a glaucomatous optic neuropathy in myopes that was not accompanied by an increased risk for elevated IOP.[2,3] In the Blue Mountains Eye Study,[2] Mitchell and co-authors reported a 4.2% prevalence of a glaucomatous optic neuropathy in low myopia patients, a 4.4% prevalence in moderate-to-high myopia patients (greater than or equal to -3D) and a 1.5% prevalence in non-myopic eyes. Daubs and Crick[3] found that moderate and high myopia substantially increased the risk for a glaucomatous optic neuropathy. Additionally, Leighton and Tomlinson[7] reported a significantly increased prevalence of axial myopia in patients with normal tension glaucoma compared with COAG.

Several studies have found increased susceptibility in myopic ocular hypertensive eyes.[8] However, in the Ocular Hypertension Treatment Study (OHTS),[9] myopia greater than -1D was not found to add significant risk for the onset of glaucomatous damage. Additionally, 47 of the 1,636 OHTS patients had myopia greater than or equal to -6D, and in this small group there was also no detectable increased risk (personal communication - Mae Gordon).

In 122 COAG patients, Chihara et al[10] found that severe myopia (greater than or equal to -4D), but not mild myopia, was a significant risk factor for progressive visual field loss. However, Jonas et al,[11] in a study of 1,444 eyes of 876 patients with primary or secondary COAG, found that for non-highly myopic (less than -8D) eyes, refractive error did not significantly contribute to ONH susceptibility.

In summary, although there are good data to suggest that myopic eyes may be at increased risk for developing elevated IOP and may have optic nerve heads that are more susceptible to developing glaucomatous damage at all levels of IOP, these data are not conclusive. However, they are sufficient to support lowering target pressures in moderate to high myopes with glaucoma at least through an initial period of care.

REFERENCES

1. David R, Zangwill LM, Tessler Z, Yassur Y. The correlation between intraocular pressure and refractive status. Arch Ophthalmol. 1985;103:1812-1815.

2. Mitchell P, Hourihan F, Sandbach J, Wang JJ. The relationship between glaucoma and myopia. The Blue Mountains Eye Study. Ophthalmology. 1999;106:2010-2015.

3. Daubs JG, Crick RP. Effect of refractive error on the risk of ocular hypertension and open angle glaucoma. Trans Ophthalmol Soc UK. 1981;101:121-126.

4. Bengtsson B. Some factors affecting the distribution of intraocular pressures in a population. Acta Ophthalmol. 1972;50:33-46.

5. Bellezza AJ, Hart RT, Burgoyne CF. The optic nerve head as a biomechanical structure: initial finite element modeling. Invest Ophthalmol Vis Sci. 2000;41:2991-3000.

6. Jonas JB, Berenshtein E, Holbach L. Lamina cribrosa thickness and spatial relationships between intraocular space and cerebrospinal fluid space in highly myopic eyes. Invest Ophthalmol Vis Sci. 2004;45:2660-2665.

7. Leighton DA, Tomlinson A. Ocular tension and axial length of the eyeball in open-angle glaucoma and low tension glaucoma. Br J Ophthalmol.1973;57:499-502.

8. Perkins ES, Phelps CD. Open angle glaucoma, ocular hypertension, low-tension glaucoma, and refraction. Arch Ophthalmol. 1982;100:1464-1467.

9. Kass MA, Heuer DK, Higginbotham EJ, Johnson CA, Keltner JL, Miller JP, Parrish RK, Wilson MR, Gordon MO. The Ocular Hypertension Treatment Study: a randomized trial determines that topical ocular hypotensive medication delays or prevents the onset of primary open-angle glaucoma. Arch Ophthalmol. 2002;120:701-713.

10. Chihara E, Liu X, Dong J, Takashima Y, Akimoto M, Hangai M, Kuriyama S, Tanihara H, Hosoda M, Tsukahara S. Severe myopia as a risk factor for progressive visual field loss in primary open-angle glaucoma. Ophthalmologica. 1997;211:66-71.

11. Jonas JB, Martus P, Budde WM. Anisometropia and degree of optic nerve damage in chronic open-angle glaucoma. Am J Ophthalmol. 2002;134:547-551.

Question 26

Is sleep apnea a risk factor for glaucoma?

Parag A. Gokhale

I believe the answer is Yes. However there are no case controlled studies to conclusively say that sleep apnea is a risk factor for glaucoma. The evidence consists primarily of case series and mechanistic theories.

Case Series:

Daniel Mojon and colleagues at the University of Bern have looked at the association of sleep apnea and glaucoma in two different populations.[1,2] They looked for the prevalence of glaucoma in a population of sleep disorder patients, and in another study they looked for the prevalence of sleep disorders in glaucoma patients.[1,2] They evaluated 114 patients undergoing polysomnography (sleep studies). Sixty-nine patients were diagnosed with sleep apnea. Five of these patients were found to have glaucoma.[1] They also looked at thirty primary open angle glaucoma patients and found that six of these patients had sleep apnea.[2]

Dennis Marcus and colleagues at the Medical College of Georgia evaluated normal tension glaucoma patients and suspects for sleep disorders. We found a high proportion of sleep disorders in normal tension glaucoma patients versus cataract patient controls.[3]

Mechanistic Possibilities:

The cause of glaucomatous optic neuropathy is not known, but the major theories include mechanical damage from intraocular pressure and/or ischemic damage. Ischemic damage may be related in part to abnormal blood flow autoregulation.[4] Sleep apnea associated glaucoma is more likely due to vascular pathology.

Sleep apnea is defined as repeated episodes of cessation of airflow with sleep.[5] With repeated apneic events the patient suffers nocturnal hypoxemia and hypercarbia.[5] Sleep apnea has been associated with many vascular effects including hypertension, congestive heart failure, myocardial infarction, and stroke.[5] Sleep apnea may be related to cases of anterior ischemic optic neuropathy.[6]

Sleep apnea is known to be associated with cerebral hypoxemia.[7] This process may be occurring at the optic nerve. With sleep apnea there are repeated events of hypoxemia and hypercarbia possibly leading to repeated episodes of decreased oxygenation to the optic nerve and disruption of blood flow autoregulation. This could lead to glaucomatous optic neuropathy.

The range of intrathoracic pressure fluctuations in sleep apnea in theory could cause elevations and fluctuations of intraocular pressure. However the initial evidence does not support elevated intraocular pressure as a mechanism in sleep apnea.[8]

Why is it important to determine an association between sleep apnea and glaucoma? At present we only have one proven way of treating glaucoma, and that is lowering intraocular pressure. Many cases of obstructive sleep apnea can be treated with positive airflow at night.[5] If there is a sleep apnea associated glaucoma, positive airflow may provide an additional treatment for this.

At present the evidence is suggestive but does not prove that sleep apnea is a risk factor for glaucoma. In order to prove this we need a clinical trial with age and weight matched controls. Some measure of blood flow and intraocular pressure would be helpful to determine possible mechanisms of this type of glaucoma.

REFERENCES

1. Mojon DS, Hess CW, Goldblum D, Fleischhauer J, Koerner F, Bassetti C, Mathis J. High prevalence of glaucoma in patients with sleep apnea syndrome. Ophthalmology, 1999; 106(5): 1009-12.

2. Mojon DS, Hess CW, Goldblum D, Böhnke M, Körner F, Mathis J. Primary open-angle glaucoma is associated with sleep apnea syndrome. Ophthalmologica, 2000; 214(2): 115-8.

3. Marcus DM, Costarides AP, Gokhale P, Papastergiou GI, Miller JJ, Johnson MH, Chaudhary BA. Sleep Disorders: A Risk Factor For Normal-Tension Glaucoma? J. Glaucoma, 2001; 10(3):177-83.

4. Anderson DR. Introductory comments on blood flow autoregulation in the optic nerve head and vascular risk factors in glaucoma. Survey of Ophthalmology, 1999; 43 Suppl 1:S5-9.

5. Chervin RD, Guilleminault C. Obstructive Sleep Apnea and Related Disorders. Neurologic Clinics, 1996; 14(3): 583-609.

6. Hayreh SS. Acute Ischemic Disorders of the Optic Nerve. Pathogenesis, clinical manifestations and management. Ophthalmol Clin North Am, 1996; 9: 407-42.

7. Hayakawa T, Terashima M, Kayukawa Y, Ohta T, Okada T. Changes in Cerebral Oxygenation and Hemodynamics during Obstructive Sleep Apneas. Chest, 1996; 109(4):916-21.

8. Goldblum D, Mathis J, Bohnke M, Bassetti C, Hess CW, Gugger M, Mojon DS. Nocturnal measurements of intraocular pressure in patients with normal-tension glaucoma and sleep apnea syndrome. Klinische Monatsblatter fur Augenheilkunde, 2000;. 216(5):246-9.

Question 27

What is the importance of IOP fluctuation in glaucoma?

Remo Susanna Jr.

Roberto M. Vessani

Primary open-angle glaucoma generally is managed by decreasing the intraocular pressure (IOP) to a level that the physician believes will prevent further glaucomatous damage. However, in a significant proportion of patients, the visual fields continue to deteriorate in spite of office pressures within the range of normal values.[1-2] It has been suggested that the progressive damage in some cases could be caused by peaks of IOP or a variability of diurnal IOP not detected by tonometry during office hours.[3-5] This has prompted clinicians to monitor the IOP more closely with diurnal tension curves (DTC) or by home tonometry. [6,7]

The importance of peaks and diurnal variation of IOP as risk factors to glaucomatous progression has been well established. Stewart et al.[8] demonstrated that a low variance in IOP over time is important in preserving visual function in advanced glaucoma. In another study, the only IOP parameter that correlated with visual field outcome was the magnitude of IOP fluctuation in normal-tension glaucoma eyes.[9] Zeimer et al.[4] found that 29% of patients with progressive visual field loss had IOP peaks during home tonometry compared with 5% of patients with stable visual fields. Martinez-Belló et al.[10] found that the peak intraocular pressure of patients who progressed was significantly different from those who remained stable in a prospective study. These authors were unable to find any difference in mean levels of intraocular pressure between the progressive and non-progressive glaucoma patients.

Evidence for the importance of pressure variations also comes from a study of Asrani et al.[7] which evaluated 64 patients with home tonometry. The large fluctuations in diurnal IOP were the most important risk factor associated with visual field loss in glaucoma patients, whereas office IOP measurements had no predictive value. The study of daily fluctuations Asrani et al.[7] , although limited by its retrospective nature and use of only one visual field for baseline, suggests that because the fluctuations of IOP per se are an independent risk factor for glaucoma progression, they may need to be treated specifically. Certain drugs or treatments could be more effective than other in dampening the fluctuations [11].

A recent report of the Advanced Glaucoma Intervention Study (AGIS) suggested that the mean IOP should be kept in the low teens and IOP peaks below 18mmHg on average to prevent further visual field deterioration in patients with moderate to advanced glaucomatous damage.[12] In this situation, it should be desirable to have the minimum long-term IOP fluctuation as possible.

The best way to access this is by performing a diurnal tension curve or monitoring the patient with home-tonometry. However, it is not feasible to determine IOP over 24 hours in most patients. Performing various IOP measurements during the day at office hours is an alternative option. It may not provide full information about IOP fluctuation such as during the nocturnal sleep period or it may not detect peaks that occurs in different times in different days, but it is more accessible than 24 hours curve.

The Water Drinking test (WDT) is another option. There is a significantly correlation between the IOP peaks in the DTC and WDT in both groups.[14] Although the water-drinking test has been shown to be a poor tool to diagnose glaucoma[13], this test has been proposed[15] as an indirect measurement of outflow facility to compare the intraocular pressure responses of an individual patient to different IOP-lowering drugs. The mechanism of IOP elevation after water drinking remains unclear. However, the ability of the eye to recover from a transient rise of intraocular pressure secondary to water ingestion is related to the pressure dependence of aqueous humor outflow, the so called outflow facility. Low facility of outflow seems to account, at least in part, for the instability and larger 24 hour IOP variations in glaucoma patients. A treatment that improves the facility of outflow might show less IOP variation in response to a water challenge, and also a less IOP variation during the day.

REFERENCES

1. Schulzer M, Mikelberg FS, Drance SM. Some observations on the relation between intraocular pressure and the progression of glaucomatous visual field loss. Br J Ophthalmol, 1987;71:486-488.

2. O´Brien C, Schwartz B, Takamoto T, Wu DC. Intraocular pressure and the rate of visual field loss in chronic open-angle glaucoma. Am J Ophthalmol, 1991;111:491-500.

3. Drance SM. Diurnal variation of intraocular pressure in treated glaucoma. Arch Ophthalmol, 1963;70:302-311.

4. Zeimer RC, Wilensky JT, Gieser DR, et al. Association between intraocular pressure peaks and progression of visual field loss. Ophthalmology, 1991; 98:64-69.

5. Katavisto M. The diurnal variations of ocular tension in glaucoma. Acta Ophthalmol, 1964;78(suppl):1-131.

6. Zeimer RC, Wilensky JT, Gieser DR, Welch DB, Mori MT, et al. Application of a self-tonometer to home tonometry. Arch Ophthalmol, 1986;104:49-53.

7. Asrani S, Zeimer R, Wilensky J, et al. Large diurnal fluctuations in intraocular pressure are an independent risk factor in patients with glaucoma. J Glaucoma, 2000;9:134-142.

8. Stewart WC, Chorak RP, Hunt HH, et al. Factors associated with visual field loss in patients with advanced glaucomatous changes in the optic nerve head. Am J Ophthalmol, 1993;116:176-181.

9. Ishida K, Yamamoto T, Kitazawa Y. clinical factors associated with progression of normal-tension glaucoma. J Glaucoma, 1998;7:372-377.

10. Martinez-Belló C, Chauhan BC, Nicolela MT, et al. Intraocular pressure and progression of glaucomatous visual field loss. Am J Ophthalmol, 2000;129:302-308.

11. Susanna JR R et al. Comparison of latanoprost with fixed – combination dorzolamide and timolol in adult patients with elevated intraocular pressure: An eight-week, randomized, open – label, parallel-group, multicenter study in Latin America Clin Ther, 2004:26: 755-768

12. The AGIS investigators. The Advanced Glaucoma Intervention Study (AGIS): 7. The relationship between control of intraocular pressure and visual field deterioration. Am J Ophthalmol, 2000;130:429-440.

13. Roth JA. Inadequate diagnostic value of the water-drinking test. Br J Ophthalmol, 1974;58:55-61.

14. Susanna R, Medeiros FA, Vessani RM. Correlation between intraocular pressure peaks in the diurnal tension curve and in the water-drinking test [ARVO Abstract]. Invest Ophthalmol Vis Sci, 2001;42:S558. Abstract nr.2995.

15. Brubaker. RF. Importance of outflow facility. In: Greve E. International Glaucoma Review. Kugler, 2001;3:10.

Question 28

What is a target pressure and how can it be calculated? (Evidence-based target pressures: how to choose them)

Paul Palmberg

Evidence based target pressures

In the original AAO Preferred Practice Pattern for POAG, published in 1989, I introduced the term "target pressure" to focus thinking on the management of glaucoma in light of the long-term outcome information available.[1-2] Now several clinical trials[3-7] have provided additional detail about the relationship between intraocular pressure and the risk of future visual field loss in patients with specific types of glaucoma.

The Advanced Glaucoma Intervention Study (AGIS) found that for patients with *POAG* and *moderate to severe damage* (average -10.5 dB Mean Deviation on Humphrey) an *optimal IOP is about 12 mm Hg* (no net progression in a group of 105 patients followed 8 years), while damage occurred at increasing frequency and severity for groups of patients in whom the IOP was higher (*Figure 1*)[3].

On the other hand, in *initially diagnosed POAG with mild damage* (average MD of -4.8 dB on Humphrey Visual Field), the Comparison of Initial Glaucoma Treatments Study (CIGTS) showed that an average 37% reduction in IOP (27 to *17.5 mm Hg*) with medication and added laser when needed, following a protocol that required advancement in treatment until the target pressure was achieved, resulted in there being no net visual field progression in 5 years.[4]

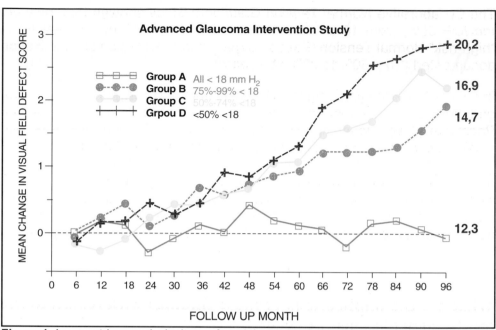

Figure 1. In a post-hoc analysis, it was found that subjects in whom the IOP at all of the semi-annual visits was below the protocol designated goal of <18 mm Hg (Group A) had no average change in AGIS visual field score (which is closely related to the Mean Deviation in Humphrey Visual Fields) during 8 years of follow up. Those in whom the IOP was <18 mm Hg on 75-99% of visits (Group B) suffered a net loss of about 2 AGIS units (equivalent to about 2.3 dB of MD). Those with 50-74% (Group C) and <50% of visits (Group D) had proportionally worse results. The mean IOP during the first 6 years of follow up was 12.3, 14.7, 16.9 and 20.2 mm Hg, respectively, for the groups.

In the Early Manifest Glaucoma Trial in Sweden,[5] in newly diagnosed patients with POAG, an average 29% reduction in IOP in POAG patients achieved a 50% reduction in relative risk of progression, with 45% of the treated and 62% of the controls progressing. The worse outcome in EMGT (average 2.2 dB MD progression in the treated, versus 3.9 dB in the untreated controls) in comparison to CIGTS (0.0 dB net worsening on treatment) might have been due to the use of a standard treatment for all, betaxolol and laser trabeculoplasty, without advancement of treatment in most cases in which the pressure was not lowered by much. An alternative explanation could have been the older age (68 versus 58) in the EMGT subjects versus those in CIGTS.

The Collaborative *Normal Tension Glaucoma* Study showed that *lowering the IOP 30%,* from 16 to *11 mm Hg,* reduced the risk of progression in "high-risk" Normal Tension Glaucoma (previous progression or split fixation documented) from 60% to 20% at 5 years[6].

In *Ocular Hypertension*[7], higher IOPs (>25 mm Hg), larger C/D, older age, and normal to thin central corneal thickness (< 555 u on Ultrasound Pachymetry) were found to be predictive of the development of POAG, with a risk of up to 36% in 5 years, and treatment that reduced the IOP about 20% reduced the relative risk of going on to glaucoma to 0.36 as much in whites and to 0.58 as much in blacks. The use of pachymetry also identified some white patients with apparent OAOH and thick corneas (about 600 microns or more) in whom a pressure of 22 mm Hg is actually about 19 mm Hg, after adjustment of the IOP for an artifact of the thick cornea, and no diagnosis of ocular hypertension or extensive work-up is indicated.[8]

What are the implications of these findings with regard to the mechanism of damage in glaucoma?

Why do patients with POAG with advanced damage and those with Normal Tension Glaucoma require a pressure below the population average to achieve the optimal result? Anderson proposed and subsequently demonstrated that some patients with glaucoma have faulty auto-regulation of blood flow at the optic nervehead.[9]. If some individuals are unable to auto-regulate optic nerve blood flow even to the extent of the difference between a normal IOP and the orbital venous pressure (which is about 8-10 mm Hg), then damage would take place in the normal pressure range. Indeed, at about 18 mm Hg 50-75% of advanced glaucoma patients progress.[6] On the other hand, at low-normal pressures no net progression was seen in the AGIS study, nor after 8 years in our study of patients operated upon with anti-metabolites.[10] (*Figure* 2). Thus, we can compensate for whatever else, besides elevated ocular pressure, is contributing to damage in these patients.

Primary Filtering Surgery with 5-FU or Mitomycin: Intraocular Pressure Control and Visual Field Data				
mm Hg	# (IOP)	MD	PSD	# fields
Pre-Op 26.1	212	-14.3	7.58	
1 Year 10.7	183	-13.6	7.59	181
2 Year 10.8	161	-12.4	7.67	117
3 Year 10.8	143	-13.3	8.18	96
4 Year 10.5	125	-13.6	8.05	71
5 Year 11.8	123	-11.9	7.68	65
6 Year 10.6	99	-13.0	9.70	47
7 Year 11.0	81	-12.6	9.34	42
8 Year 11.8	63	-12.7	8.79	22
9 Year 10.4	46	-10.7	7.42	19
10 Year 11.0	30	-12.1	8.71	13
Ishida K, E Escalona, J Schiffman, Palmberg P, ARVO 2003 Tecnique: Suner, et al, Ophthalmology 1997:104:207-214.				

Figure 2. Pre-operative and yearly post-operative intraocular pressures in a consecutive series of cases operated upon with 5-FU or Mitomycin C, and the corresponding visual field results. There was no net visual field progression for the group.

On the other hand, patients with mild, initial glaucoma damage, appear only to need a reduction to the mid-upper normal IOP level to achieve stability. It remains to be seen whether some of these patients will go on to need even lower pressures as they age, or whether such increased sensitivity to pressure develops as a consequence of allowing damage to progress. The outcome studies are summarized in *Figure 3*.

In summary, we now have quite useful guidance from clinical trials to help us choose target pressures likely to avoid visual field damage/progression, and potent medical, laser and surgical treatments to achieve our goals. Clinical judgment remains important, however, as we may need to modify our pressure goals in light of the history of the patient at hand, the effectiveness and side-effects of treatment in them, their ability to comply and social factors.

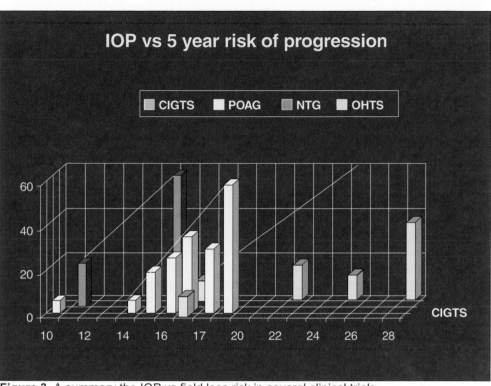

Figure 3. A summary the IOP vs field loss risk in several clinical trials.

Back to the Future

Paul Chandler said it best (AJO 1960):

- "Eyes with advanced glaucoma...require a pressure below the average normal..."

- "Eyes with limited cupping, confined to one pole of the disc, appear to withstand tension better..."

- "Eyes with a normal disc appear to withstand pressure well...over many years..."

- "The appearance of the disc may serve as an important guide to the management of glaucoma."

REFERENCES

1. Glaucoma panel. The Preferred Practice Pattern for Primary Open-Angle Glaucoma. American Academy of Ophthalmology, 1969, San Francisco, CA.

2. Chandler PA. Long-term results of glaucoma therapy. Am J Ophthalmol 1960;49:221-246.

3. The AGIS Investigators. The Advanced Glaucoma Intervention Study (AGIS). 7. The relationship between control of intraocular pressure control and visual field deterioration. Am J Ophthalmol 2000;130:429-440.

4. Lichter PR, Musch DC, Gillespie BW, Guire KE, Janz NK, Wren PA, Mills RP; CIGTS Study Group. Interim clinical outcomes in the Collaborative Initial Glaucoma Treatment Study comparing initial treatment randomized to medications or surgery. Ophthalmol 2001;108:1939-1950.

5. Heijl A, Leske MC, Bengtsson B, Hyman L, Bengtsson B, Hussein M; Early Manifest Glaucoma Trial Group. Reduction of intraocular pressure and glaucoma progression: results from the Early Manifest Glaucoma Trial. Arch Ophthalmol 2002;120:1268-1279.

6. The CNTGS Group. The effectiveness of intraocular pressure reduction in the treatment of normal-tension glaucoma. Am J Ophthalmol 1998;126:498-505.

7. Kass MA, Heuer DK, Higginbothan EJ, Johnson CA, Keltner JL, Miller JP, Parrish RK II, Wilson MR, Gordon MO. The Ocular Hypertension Treatment Study: a randomized trial determines that topical ocular hypotensive medication delays or prevents the onset of primary open-angle glaucoma. Arch Ophthalmol 2002;120:701-13.

8. Brandt JD, Beiser JA, Kass MA, Gordon MO. Central corneal thickness in the Ocular Hypertension Treatment Study (OHTS). Ophthalmology 2001;108:1779-1788.

9. Anderson DR. Introductory comments on blood flow autoregulation in the optic nerve head and vascular risk factors in glaucoma. Surv Ophthalmol 1999;43(Suppl 1):S5-S9.

10. Ishida K, Benz EE, Schiffman JC, Palmberg PF. Long-term results of primary filtering surgery with adjunctive antimetabolites. Invest Oph Vis Sci 2003;43 (Suppl):91.

Question 29

Is treatment of early glaucoma important?

Anders Heijl

IOP reduction effective

After a long period when we have become aware of the less than perfect relationship between IOP and glaucoma damage, recently published randomized trials have shed new and much needed light on the effect of IOP reduction in glaucoma. In studies with untreated control groups EMGT and CNTGS have demonstrated the effectiveness of IOP lowering, and there is now no doubt that IOP reduction reduces the progression of glaucoma damage[1,2]. Similarly OHTS showed that IOP reduction also decreases the incidence of glaucoma damage in patients with elevated IOP[3]. EMGT has provided an estimate of the magnitude of the effects, around 10% risk reduction per mmHg of IOP reduction[1,4].

Knowing the positive effects of our conventional treatment, it might be tempting to suggest maximum IOP reduction given as early as possible should be the norm in all patients regardless of the stage of the disease. But treatment is associated both with cost, side effects and inconvenience. Furthermore identification of early glaucoma is not easy, first because about 50% of patients with manifest glaucoma (with visual field defects on standard white-on-white automated perimetry) are unknown, and secondly because pushing the diagnosis towards earlier disease stage is associated with increasing numbers of patients with a false positive diagnosis, and thus also with unnecessarily reduced quality of life.

The goal of treatment

The Guidelines of the European Glaucoma Society formulate a goal for glaucoma treatment "The goal of glaucoma treatment is to maintain the patient's quality of life at a sustainable cost"[5]. This means that it is important to focus on the patient's subjective visual function now and during his remaining life time and to remember quality of life-issues, also such issues that are unrelated to visual function. Odberg et al. have shown that a glaucoma diagnosis has psychologically induced negative impact on quality of life, independent of visual function[6].

Natural history and velocity of progression

We must then take into consideration what will happen without treatment. We now have some knowledge of the natural history of manifest glaucoma. In EMGT average velocity of progression of untreated patients was a worsening of MD of −0.05 ±0.07 dB per month, or 6dB for 10 years[1]. Unfortunately inter-individual variation of the velocity of progression is very large. EMGT showed that the spectrum is very wide; some patients progressed within 6 months, others, including untreated controls, have not shown progression after 10 years. Progression velocities are shown in Figure 1. In CNTGS this variation was also very high[3]. We cannot, therefore, predict the natural history for the individual patient, but we can use our knowledge of risk factors for progression. We must also remember that the natural history is not well known for eyes with higher IOP levels (> 30mmHg).

Early treatment?

Where does this lead us regarding the question of early treatment. The latter can mean two different things: 1) initial treatment after the diagnosis, or 2. treatment early in the course of the disease.

Intial treatment

An evidence-based approach to treatment for the individual patient should initially be based on prior knowledge, i.e. the degree of damage present,

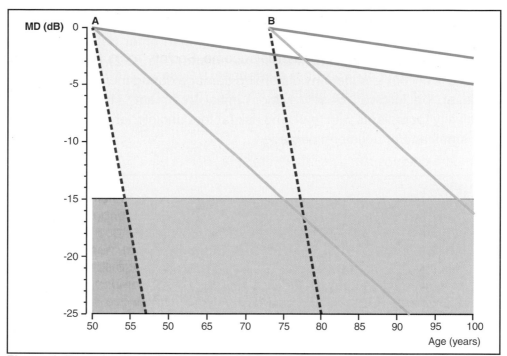

Figure. 1. Examples illustrating the natural history of glaucoma progression from the time of first (perimetric) glaucoma damage. The solid yellow lines represent approximate mean progression rates in untreatred patients EMGT (a worsening of . 6dB/10 years) and the green lines estimated best and red lines worst progression rates. It is clear from the illustration than on the average patients who first develop glaucoma damage when being followed (thus starting at MD values close to 0) would have very a good chance of not reaching serious damage (here defined as MD values worse than –15dB, grey area) even if left untreated if they are elderly (patient B). An untreated patient with manifest glaucoma damage already at 50 years of age (patient A), would, on the contrary have a large risk of serious damage during his life-time. The difference between worst (red lines) and best case scenarios is very wide however (this area is yellow for the younger patient A). Thus a good prediction cannot be made until the patient has been followed for a few years and the rate of progression determined.

IOP level, age and life expectancy. High IOP and larger damage have both been shown to be associated with more rapid progression than lower IOP and less damage[1,3]. Higher age is also a risk factor, but despite this younger patients are at higher risk for serious damage because of their longer life expectancy. Exfoliation is also a strong and independent risk factor, but there is no strong proof for other factors, e.g., cardiovascular status, corneal thickness, migraine or refraction[4].

Patients with more risk factors are likely to progress faster and should therefore be treated more vigorously initially than other patients with the same amount of damage and age/life expectancy (Figure 2). Some patients that are likely not to suffer any disturbing damage during their lifetime could, however, be followed closely without initial treatment. This should be a possibility for patients with few or no risk factors and higher age, particularly with small and/or unilateral damage.

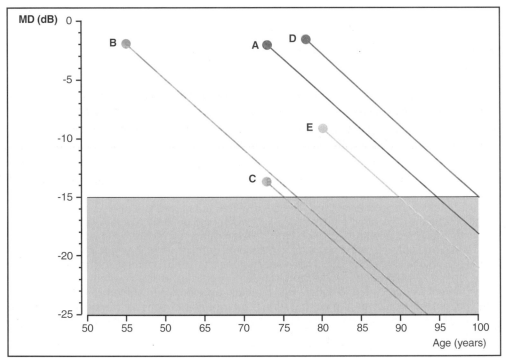

Figure 2. A patient's age, and thus life expectancy, and amount of glaucoma damage dictate whether intense treatment, or even treatment at all, is needed. Solid oblique lines represent the mean progression rate in untreated eyes in EMGT (. 6dB/10 years). A glaucoma patient detected at the average age at detection in Malmö (73 years) with mild glaucoma loss (MD = -2dB – red patient A) has a good chance to avoid subjectively disturbing damage (grey area – worse than −15dB) during his life time even if left untreated and living to a very high age. The risk is much higher if the patient is young (55 years) even with the same damage (green patient B). Most patients are detected with moderate to advanced disease at fairly high age (blue patient C), and then there is very little or no margin to serious loss, and such patients should definitely be treated immediately. The older patients (violet patient D and yellow patient E) have smaller risks of serious loss, and then follow-up without treatment may be the preferred initial approach for many patients.

Unfortunately, glaucoma patients are very often diagnosed late with very substantial damage[7], and then early i.e. undelayed treatment is almost always highly motivated.

The individual patient's rate of progression can then be assessed by threshold perimetry 3 times per year during the first 2 or 3 years. With knowledge of the rate of progression, the amount damage and the patient's age and general health, the ophthalmologist will then be able to provide the patient with the right amount of individually tailored therapy.

Treatment early in the course of the disease

Treatment early in the course of the disease, i.e. when damage is minimal or uncertain, is something entirely different. There is a lot of margin before the patient has damage that reduces the patients subjective functioning or quality of life. Generally speaking treatment early in the course of the disease is only important in patients with risk factors often in combination: high IOP values, exfoliation, young age and long life expectancy (cf. Figure 2).

Summary

With our new knowledge that IOP reduction on the average is very effective, but also that the natural history of glaucoma is highly variable between patients, we should seek to tailor glaucoma treatment to patients' individual needs.

Early treatment is often, but not always, appropriate. Only in younger patients with important risk factors is treatment early in the course of the disease always needed.

From a public health point of view, it is my opinion that it may be more fruitful to try to identify some of the many patients with well established but undiagnosed disease, than to strive for very early diagnosis in glaucoma suspects.

REFERENCES

1. Heijl A, Leske MC, Bengtsson B, Hyman L, Bengtsson Boel, Hussein M, Early Manifest Glaucoma Trial Group. Reduction of intraocular pressure and glaucoma progression. Results from the Early Manifest Glaucoma Trial. Arch Ophthalmol 2002;120:1268-1279.

2. Kass MA, Heuer DK, Higginbotham EJ, et al. The Ocular Hypertension Treatment Study: a randomized trial determines that topical ocular hypotensive medication delays or prevents the onset of primary open-angle glaucoma. Arch Ophthalmol 2002;120:701-713.

3. Collaborative Normal-Tension Glaucoma Study Group. The effectiveness of intraocular pressure reduction in the treatment of normal-tension glaucoma. Am J Ophthalmol 1998;126:498-505.

4. Leske MC. Heijl A, Hussein M, Begtsson B, Hyman L. Komaroff E, Early Manifest Glaucoma Trial Group. Factors for glaucoma progression and the effect of treatment: the Early Manifest Glaucoma Trial. Arch Ophthalmol. 2003;121:48-56.

5. European Glaucoma Society. Terminology and Guidelines for Glaucoma, 2nd edition p. 3-3, Editrice DOGMA S.r.l., Savona, 2003

6. Odberg T, Jakobsen JE, Hultgren SJ, Halseide R. The impact of glaucoma on the quality of life of patients in Norway. I. Results from a self-administered questionnaire. Acta Ophthalmol Scand 2001;79:116-120.

7. Grødum K, Heijl A, Bengtsson B. A comparison of glaucoma patients identified through mass screening and in routine clinical practice. Acta Ophthalmol Scand 2002;80:627-631.

Question 30

What is the role of rate of progression in the management of glaucoma?

Erik L. Greve

The aim of glaucoma management is to prevent reduced Quality of Vision (QoV) and Quality of Life (QoL). Reduced QoV will be experienced in the presence of advanced binocular visual field defects or through side effects of medications. Reduced QoL will be experienced by reduced QoV, by the knowledge of having glaucoma, ·by side-effects of medications or other forms of treatment, by frequent visits to the doctor and high costs of treatment[1].

Treatment of glaucoma can be based on RISK or on FACT[2]. The most important FACT is an individual Rate of Progression (RoP) that is likely to affect the patients QoV within his expected lifespan. All treatment should preferably be based on this FACT unless reduced QoV is already present or the present RISK of developing reduced QoV is so high that establishing RoP is unacceptable*. One of the major reasons for using FACT as a guidance for glaucoma management is the tremendous and <u>unpredictable inter-individual variation in RoP</u>. Whenever it is possible (patient, stage of disease, instrumentation, cost) to establish RoP this should be our preference also because RoP is usually slow[3,4].

---

* Note that RISK is NOT the risk of conversion from ocular hypertension to glaucoma but the RISK of reduced QoV.

Treatment based on FACT presumes that:

- we know at which stage of functional or structural loss reduced QoV will be noticed.
- we know the approximate expected lifespan of the patient.
- we can safely and practically measure RoP within a reasonable timespan.

At the moment of writing no consensus exists on the <u>amount of damage that will cause reduced QoV</u>[5,6]. Until appropriate studies have been performed one could arbitrarily – and on the safe side – use a level of visual field that allows the patient to drive without problems. Paracentral or centrocoecal defects may cause reduced QoV in an earlier stage.

The <u>expected lifespan</u> of the patient can be deducted from actuarial tables. In the individual case this will never be ideal and it seems prudent to remain on the safe side by expecting a reasonably long lifespan

In the EMGT the RoP expressed as change of median untreated deviation in dB/month was 0.05 (0.60/dB/yr; 6 dB/10 yrs; 12 dB/20 yrs). This assumes more or less a linear approach to RoP. No doubt the <u>calculation of RoP</u> will be refined in the near future. In the mean time the crude MD/time is a reasonable option.

Establishing RoP requires at least 5 repeated measurements. The time-span which is needed to establish RoP will depend on frequency of visual field examinations. When 3 visual fields are made in the first years – as has been suggested – RoP could already be known after two years.

It is realized that this frequency deviates from current practice. Reimbursement and other practical problems may come up. It will therefore be necessary to demonstrate not only that QoV reduction can be predicted and prevented but also that management based on RoP and QoV is cost-effective.

In this context the Number Needed to Treat (NNT) is of interest[2,7,8]. The NNT is the number of patients needed to treat in order to prevent one event to happen. The NNT is the inverse of the Absolute Risk Reduction (ARR). If we use FACT (= establishing RoP) as the foundation for our glaucoma-management-decisions we need to treat only ONE patient: NNT =

1. If we use RISK we unfortunately will have to treat a number of patients (depending on end point) in order to prevent deterioration in that ONE patient. It seems quite clear that whenever possible it is our preference to treat only that ONE patient by using RoP, QoV and expected lifespan.

In the OHTS the NNT in order to prevent conversion to early visual field defects is 42. Consequently the NNT in order to prevent reduced QoV is much greater (exact number not known). In terms of QOL and costs for all those patients it is questionable whether one should treat OHT (IOP<= 30 mmHg) without additional strong risk factors that reduce the NNT considerably[9,10].

In the EMGT the NNT for preventing progression in patients with early glaucoma is 5-6. Given the slow mean RoP the NNT to prevent reduced QoV will again be much greater. Here too it may be preferable to treat only the patients who really need treatment and to follow the others who do not need it, carefully[4,10].

REFERENCES

1. Odberg T, Jakobsen JE, Hultgren SJ, Halseide R. The impact of glaucoma on the quality of life of patients in Norway. I. Results from a self-administered questionnaire. Acta Ophthalmol, 2001; 79: 116-120.

2. Greve EL, Hitchings RA Management of Glaucoma based on rate of progression and quality of life; lessons from the RCT's. Int. Glaucoma Review, 2002; 4(3): 448-451.

3. Anderson DR, Drance SM, Schulzer M. Collaborative Normal-Tension Glaucoma Study Group. Natural history of Normal Tension Glaucoma. Ophthalmology, 2001; 108: 247-253.

4. Heijl A, et al Reduction of intraocular pressure and glaucoma progression: results from the Early Manifest Glaucoma Trial. Arch Ophthalmol, 2002; 120: 1268-1279.

5. Mills RA. Correlation of quality of life with clinical symptoms and signs at the time of glaucoma diagnosis. Trans Am Ophthalmol Soc, 1998;96:753-812.

6. Viswanathan AC, McNaught AI, Poinoosawmy D, Fontana L, Crabb DP, Fitzke FW, Hitchings RA. Severity and stability of glaucoma: patient perception compared with objective measurement. Arch Ophthalmol, 1999; 117: 450-454.

7. Coleman AL. Applying evidence-based medicine in ophthalmic practice. Am J Ophthalmol, 2002; 134: 599-601.

8. Wilson R. NNT. Treatment for ocular hypertension and early glaucoma: how much benefit and is it worth the cost? Int Glaucoma Review, 2003; 5(1): 10 + comment by EL Greve and RA Hitchings.

9. Kass MA, et al The Ocular Hypertension Treatment Study: a randomized trial determines that topical ocular hypotensive medication delays or prevents the onset of primary open-angle glaucoma. Arch Ophthalmol, 2002; 120: 701-713.

10. Lichter PR. Glaucoma clinical trials asn what they mean for our patients. Am J Ophthalmol, 2003; 136: 136-145.

Question 31

How can one optimally follow patients with end-stage glaucoma and advanced visual field loss?

Ivan Goldberg

Glaucomatous optic neuropathy manifests structural damage before detectable functional loss. (Figure 1.) Early loss therefore is best diagnosed structurally including localized or sectoral erosion of the neural rim, increase in depth and/or extent of cupping and later development or increase in peripapillary atrophy and nasal displacement of blood vessels.

Good glaucoma management demands intelligent use of time, which in turn requires us to set baseline measurements for structure and function and to monitor whether or not these are stable (meaning treatment is succeeding) or they are deteriorating (meaning treatment is failing). Structure can be documented by careful description and drawing of the disc, photographs (preferably stereoscopic) and/or sophisticated imaging technology such as the HRT, GDx or OCT. Recording cup to disc ratios by colour and contour may be useful too, as long as absolute disc size is taken into account – larger discs normally have larger cups. Functional status needs quantitative perimetric techniques. Currently these are subjective.

Advanced loss means the optic disc is "cupped out" with extensive visual field loss. At this stage of damage, the cup almost fills the disc and there is little neural rim remaining to observe or to measure; careful ophthalmoscopy will only permit detection of peripapillary nerve fibre layer haemorrhages, not any additional erosion of the neural rim remnant. It is on the perimetric results that we now rely.

145

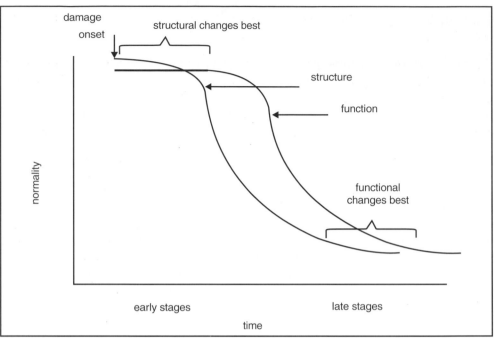

Figure 1. Schematic representation of conceptual time course of structural versus functional damage in glaucoma. Initially structural changes can be detected most sensitively; at moderate levels of damage, both structural and functional changes can be detected; in advanced disease, with structural damage at its end-point, it is functional progression that can be assessed most effectively. (Adapted from RN Weinreb)

A tiny remaining central tunnel of vision cannot be followed accurately with standard visual fields – the 24-2 and 30-2 programs of the Humphrey, or their equivalents with other perimeters, have a central density of tested points of 6-degrees. With advanced loss, the entire remaining central field may lie within 10 degrees. For central visual function, it is the 10-2 program with its 2-degree tested point density that we need to use. As always, analysis of both the extent and the sensitivity of the remaining visual field are critical to determine whether or not progressive damage is occurring.

Because subjective perimetry is so variable even for the most reliable patients, and because that variability increases with more advanced disease, if progression is suspected, confirmation by at least one repeated visual field test is mandatory. It may be necessary to achieve confirmation with two follow-up assessments. This is particularly the case if a decision to proceed to surgery, or repeat surgery is based on apparent perimetric progression.

If there is a temporal crescent remaining, perimetric testing may need to be unconventional - either 30-60 static bands should be assessed (accuracy falls off considerably), kinetic perimeters employed, or even Bjerrum or confrontation techniques used. Although such peripheral testing is more qualitative than quantitative, it can be helpful in determining stability or not.

At these stages of the disease, patients can often provide useful subjective impressions of visual function. Any complaints of progressive visual disability must be taken seriously, even if perimetric analysis appears to be unchanged.

In patients with advanced glaucomatous damage, therefore, assessment of the extent and depth of functional loss becomes more helpful than evaluation of disc structure. Because such assessment relies currently on subjective methods, repeated testing is vital if therapeutic decisions are to be based reliably on these results.

Question 32

How should normal tension glaucoma be managed?

Marcelo T. Nicolela

Initially, I would like to state that I don't consider normal tension glaucoma (NTG) a different disease entity from primary open angle glaucoma (POAG), but just as one spectrum of a group of optic neuropathies that produce typical optic disc and visual field defects, associated with open angle on gonioscopy and variable levels of intraocular pressure (IOP). Nevertheless, the management of patients with NTG is somewhat different than that of patients with elevated IOP, since glaucoma therapy is based on reduction of IOP.

The first question to consider is whether IOP reduction has a positive outcome impact in these patients. Recently published data from the Collaborative Normal-Tension Glaucoma Study (CNTGS)[1,2] and from the Early Manifest Glaucoma Trial (EMGT)[3], in which approximately 50% of the patients enrolled had normal IOP, showed that patients randomized to IOP reduction had better outcome than patients randomized to observation only, proving the benefits of IOP lowering in patients with normal IOP.

There are, however, other interesting questions regarding the management of patients with NTG. Should every NTG patient be treated? In order to answer this question, we need to know the natural history of NTG, the potential risk factors associated to disease progression and side effects of therapy. The CNTGS showed that approximately 50% of patients with NTG failed to show disease progression when observed for at least 5 years, and, moreover, several patients who progressed did so at a very slow rate. Female gender and presence of optic disc hemorrhages or migraine were significantly associated to disease progression.[4] It is, therefore, reasonable to observe NTG patients closely without treatment, particularly those with

149

milder disease. Observation and monitoring would allow the determination of whether the patient has a more progressive form of the disease, warranting treatment. I would consider starting treatment soon after diagnosis in patients with more advanced disease, with some of the previously identified risk factors for progression, such as migraine or optic disc hemorrhages, or with IOP at the higher end of normality.

How should we set target pressures for NTG patients? Unfortunately, the information available in the literature on this issue is scarce. In the CNTGS, 30% IOP reduction was chosen, but we don't know if 20% would be enough or if 40% would be better. There is always a price to pay depending on how aggressive we want to be, as lower target IOP might mean multiple drugs, laser or surgical therapies. I set the target between 20 to 40% IOP reduction, depending on how advanced the disease is and other associated factors such as age, health status and additional risk factors.

What is the role of diurnal IOP curves in diagnosing NTG? Since I don't consider NTG a different disease from POAG, I don't perform diurnal tension curves in every patient with NTG. It is important, however, to have good information regarding IOP fluctuation before starting treatment. In these cases, as well as for most POAG patients, my goal is to obtain several IOP measurements before starting treatment, either on the same day or during several visits at different times of the day.

What is the role of neuro-imaging in NTG? There are still controversies in this area.[5,6] I reserve investigation with neuro-imaging for NTG patients with no correlation between visual field and optic disc damage (worse visual field status than what would be expected from the disc status), with vertically aligned visual field defects, with optic disc pallor in excess of cupping or with reduced visual acuity of unexplained reason.

What should be the first line agents in NTG? Ocular hypotensive lipids are probably the best first line agents in NTG for several reasons: better IOP response than other agents; greater chances of achieving low target IOP; few systemic side effects, particularly no cardiovascular adverse effects, and flatter diurnal IOP fluctuation.[7]

How to monitor NTG patients? These patients should be monitored similarly to other POAG patients. There are, however, few particularities to consider. NTG patients have frequently visual field defects close to fixation and, in that case, should be monitored with visual field strategies that have a good concentration of points in the central area, such as the C10-2 test of the Humphrey Field Analyzer. Patients with NTG tend to have optic disc hemorrhages more frequently than ordinary POAG patients, and particular care should be taken at every visit in the examination of the optic disc to rule out disc hemorrhages.[8]

When to consider other treatment modalities for NTG patients, such as calcium channel blockers, neuroprotection, and ginkgo? There is a paucity of data regarding the long-term effects of treatments other than IOP reduction in glaucoma.[9,10,11,12] I have used calcium channel blockers in patients who continue to progress despite maximal IOP reduction, particularly in those patients with evidence of vasospastic disease (migraine, Raynaud's phenomenon). In these cases, I always involve the patient's internist in the decision and monitor blood pressure very carefully, since these agents can cause a significant decrease in blood pressure, which could lead to decreased optic disc perfusion.

REFERENCES

1. The effectiveness of intraocular pressure reduction in the treatment of normal-tension glaucoma. Collaborative Normal-Tension Glaucoma Study Group. Am J Ophthalmol, 1998. 126(4): p. 498-505.

2. Comparison of glaucomatous progression between untreated patients with normal-tension glaucoma and patients with therapeutically reduced intraocular pressures. Collaborative Normal-Tension Glaucoma Study Group. Am J Ophthalmol, 1998. 126(4): p. 487-97.

3. Heijl, A., et al., Reduction of intraocular pressure and glaucoma progression: results from the Early Manifest Glaucoma Trial. Arch Ophthalmol, 2002. 120(10): p. 1268-79.

4. Drance, S., D.R. Anderson, and M. Schulzer, Risk factors for progression of visual field abnormalities in normal- tension glaucoma. Am J Ophthalmol, 2001. 131(6): p. 699-708.

5. Greenfield, D.S., et al., The cupped disc. Who needs neuroimaging? Ophthalmology, 1998. 105(10): p. 1866-74.

6. Ahmed, II, et al., Neuroradiologic screening in normal-pressure glaucoma: study results and literature review. J Glaucoma, 2002. 11(4): p. 279-86.

7. Drance, S.M., A. Crichton, and R.P. Mills, Comparison of the effect of latanoprost 0.005% and timolol 0.5% on the calculated ocular perfusion pressure in patients with normal-tension glaucoma. Am J Ophthalmol, 1998. 125(5): p. 585-92.

8. Kitazawa, Y., S. Shirato, and T. Yamamoto, Optic disc hemorrhage in low-tension glaucoma. Ophthalmology, 1986. 93(6): p. 853-7.

9. Rainer, G., et al., A double masked placebo controlled study on the effect of nifedipine on optic nerve blood flow and visual field function in patients with open angle glaucoma. Br J Clin Pharmacol, 2001. 52(2): p. 210-2.

10. Quaranta, L., et al., Effect of Ginkgo biloba extract on preexisting visual field damage in normal tension glaucoma. Ophthalmology, 2003. 110(2): p. 359-62; discussion 362-4.

11. Rhee, D.J., et al., Complementary and alternative medicine for glaucoma. Surv Ophthalmol, 2001. 46(1): p. 43-55.

12. Kitazawa, Y., H. Shirai, and F.J. Go, The effect of Ca2(+) -antagonist on visual field in low-tension glaucoma. Graefes Arch Clin Exp Ophthalmol, 1989. 227(5): p. 408-12.

Question 33

Is laser iridotomy indicated in the management of pigmentary dispersion syndrome?

M. Bruce Shields

The constellation of clinical findings, which leads to the diagnosis of pigmentary glaucoma (PG), has puzzled clinicians and scientists since Sugar and Barbour described the condition in 1949[1]. Why does it occur predominantly in young, myopic men? What is the mechanism of the pigment dispersion that is seen on the cornea as Krukenberg's spindle, on the iris stroma and especially in the trabecular meshwork? What do the spoke-like, mid-peripheral transillumination iris defects tell us about this mechanism? Why do these patients develop glaucoma? And, most importantly, how can this information guide us to better ways of treating patients with pigmentary glaucoma?

During the final quarter of the twentieth century, answers were offered for many of these questions. Outflow obstruction appears to begin with an accumulation of pigment granules in the trabecular meshwork. Over time, this partially reversible stage evolves into one that is less reversible, as trabecular endothelial cells engulf the pigment and eventually detach from the trabecular beams, which subsequently collapse[2,3].

In 1979, Campbell[4] proposed that anterior packets of lens zonules rub against iris pigment epithelium, leading to the dispersion of pigment, referred to as pigment dispersion syndrome (PDS), with subsequent PG developing in a percentage of these patients. Campbell further postulated (in his *1991*American Glaucoma Society Lecture, honoring Dr Sugar) that the rubbing is due to the posterior bowing of the peripheral iris and that this contour of the iris can be converted to a planar configuration with a laser

153

peripheral iridotomy (LPI). Although this observation has been confirmed by Karickhoff[5] and by the clinical experience of many surgeons, preliminary reports on the long-term benefit of LPI in patients with PG have been conflicting[6,7]. In this chapter, we will consider the evidence for a role of LPI in PG and an approach to this treatment modality in our clinical practice.

A role for the dispersed pigment in the mechanism of the glaucoma was suggested by the early work of Sugar and Barbour[1]. Light and electron microscopic studies confirmed this theory, showing pigment granules in the intertrabecular spaces in the relatively early stages of the disorder, with loss of the trabecular meshwork cells and collapse of trabecular beams in the latter stages[2,3]. The mechanism of the pigment dispersion was elucidated by Campbell[4], who provided evidence for a rubbing between lens zonules and iris pigment epithelium, with release of pigment granules. The rubbing results from posterior bowing of the peripheral iris, which in turn is due to a reverse pressure gradient between the anterior and posterior chambers. Studies with ultrasound biomicroscopy (UBM) have shown a more posterior than normal insertion of the iris in patients with PDS[8] and have suggested that the reverse pressure gradient is due to a reverse pupillary block, in which aqueous humor is "pumped" into the anterior chamber by movement of the iris, but is prevented from flowing backward due to the valve effect of the iris against the lens[9]. However, it has been the observations associated with LPI that provides the strongest support fort the latter concept[5]. At the moment of iris

penetration, when performing an LPI in a patient with PG, the surgeon may observe aqueous flowing backward through the iridotomy into the posterior chamber, and the contour of the peripheral iris changes from concave to planar. Ultrasound biomicroscopic studies have supported the change in iris configuration[10,11], as well as a decrease in iridolenticular contact[11], following LPI.

While LPI in patients with PG has clearly been shown to eliminate the reverse pressure gradient and posterior bowing of the peripheral iris, it is not known whether this

alteration in the contour of the iris favorably alters the long-term course of the IOP in these patients. If such a favorable outcome were proven to be the case, we would have a very effective method for treating PG at the early, initiating stage of the disorder, much as we have for pupillary block angle-closure glaucoma. To date, however, despite the introduction of LPI for PG more than a decade ago, there has not been a large, prospective, controlled, longitudinal study to prove the efficacy of LPI in the long-term IOP course in PG patients.

Gandolfi and Vecchi[6] reported a prospective study of 21 individuals with PDS, who received an LPI in one eye and were noted to have an IOP rise (more than 5 mmHg) in one (4.7%) treated eye and eleven (52.3%) fellow eyes during a 2-year follow-up. However, in a retrospective study of 17 patients with PDS or PG, treated with unilateral

LPI, Wang, Liebmann and Ritch[7] found no significant long-term IOP reduction in iridotomy eyes, compared to medically treated fellow eyes.

At the present time, therefore, there is only indirect evidence, at best, that an LPI may be beneficial in managing the patient with pigmentary glaucoma. What then should the Ophthalmologist recommend to his or her patients with this condition? First, we must understand the theory of why it might be beneficial and then determine in which patients it may be indicated.

Unlike LPI for pupillary-block angle-closure glaucoma, in which we anticipate a prompt reduction in IOP, this should not be expected in the patient with pigmentary glaucoma. If anything, the pressure may initially rise, possibly due to further pigment dispersion, and this may persist for several months before a gradual improvement in IOP is seen. The theory behind this clinical observation is that, by eliminating the reverse pupillary block and hence the rubbing between iris and lens zonules, LPI reduces the continued liberation of pigment granules. Over time (probably years), this reduction of pigment accumulation in the trabecular meshwork allows improved outflow, unless irreversible damage has already occurred.

If LPI is to benefit the patient with PG, it would, in theory, need to be done before significant damage has occurred to the trabecular meshwork (much less to the optic nerve). Relatively older patients, who have had the glaucoma for many years, are less likely to benefit from the iridotomy. The best candidate would be the person with PDS, who is destined to eventually develop IOP elevation and PG. Unfortunately, however, we currently have no means of predicting which patients with PDS will go on to develop PG. One large study has suggested that the risk of converting is approximately 10% at 5 years and 15% and 15 years[12]. To treat all patients with PDS, therefore, is not advisable. The best approach may be to follow each PDS patient closely as a "pigmentary glaucoma suspect," watching for an upward trend in the IOP, and to then discuss with that patient the pros and cons of a prophylactic LPI. The best we can tell them at this time is that the risk of the procedure is relatively low and that it might improve their long-term course.

Hopefully, the appropriate clinical trial will one day be performed to establish the role of LPI in patients with PG. Until then, we will have to use our best clinical judgment, based on the evidence that is presently available.

REFERENCES

1. Sugar HS, Barbour FA. Pigmentary glaucoma. A rare clinical entity. Am J Ophthalmol, 1949; 32: 90-92.

2. Richardson TM, Hutchinson BT, Grant WM. The outflow tract in pigmentary glaucoma: a light and electron microscopic study. Arch Ophthalmol, 1977; 95: 1015-25.

3. Kampik A, Green WR, Quigley HA, et al. Scanning and transmission electron microscopic studies of two cases of pigment dispersion syndrome. Am J Ophthalmol, 1981; 91: 573-87.

4. Campbell DG. Pigmentary dispersion and glaucoma. A new theory. Arch Ophthalmol, 1979; 97: 1667-1672.

5. Karickhoff JR. Pigment dispersion syndrome and pigmentary glaucoma: a new mechanism concept, a new treatment, and a new technique. Ophthalmic Surg, 1992; 23: 269-77.

6. Gandolfi SA, Vecchi M. Effect of a YAG laser iridotomy on the intraocular pressue in pigment dispersion. Ophthalmology, 1996; 103: 1693-1695.

7. Wang JC, Liebermann JM, Ritch R. Long-term outcome of argon iridotomy in pigment dispersion syndrome. Invest Ophthalmol Vis Sci (Suppl), 2001; 42: s560.

8. Sokol J, Stegman Z, Liebman JM, et al. Location of the iris insertion in pigment dispersion syndrome. Ophthalmology, 1996; 103: 289-93.

9. Pavlin CJ, Macken P, Trope G, et al. Ultrasound biomicroscopic features of pigmentary glaucoma. Can J Ophthalmol, 1994; 29: 187-192.

10. Pavlin CJ, Macken P, Trope G, et al. Accomodation and iridotomy in the pigment dispersion syndrome. Ophthalmic Surg & Lasers, 1996; 27: 113-20.

11. Breingan PJ, Esaki K, Ishikawa H, et al. Iridolenticular contact decreases following laser iridotomy for pigment dispersion syndrome. Arch Ophthalmol, 1999;117: 325-328.

12. Siddiqui Y, Ten Hulzen RD, Cameron JD, et al. What is the risk of developing pigmentary glaucoma from pigment dispersion syndrome? Am J Ophthalmol, 2003; 135: 794-799.

Question 34

Why is intraocular pressure difficult to control in exfoliation syndrome?

Robert Ritch

Vincent Hugo

Exfoliation syndrome (XFS) is overall the most common identifiable cause of glaucoma, accounting for the majority of cases in some countries, and causing both open-angle glaucoma and angle-closure glaucoma.[1] Glaucoma occurs more commonly in eyes with exfoliation syndrome (XFS) than in those without it. Most series indicate that about 25% of patients with XFS have elevated intraocular pressure (IOP) and one-third of these have glaucomatous damage. This is approximately 6 times the chance of finding elevated IOP in eyes without XFS.[2-5] In persons with XFS, the risk of developing glaucoma is cumulative over time, having approximately a 40% chance of either having initially or developing ocular hypertension or glaucoma within ten years, approximately a ten-fold increased risk when compared to the general population.[6] Both age and elevated IOP increase the risk of conversion of OHT to glaucoma and persons with elevated IOP and XFS are more likely to progress to glaucomatous damage than are those with elevated IOP without XFS.[7,8] The severity of the disease is reflected in the fact that the proportion of patients with XFS shows a steady increase when measured in cohorts with open-angle glaucoma without optic nerve damage, in those with damage, in those undergoing surgery, and in those with absolute glaucoma.

Glaucoma in XFS has a more serious clinical course and worse prognosis than does primary open-angle glaucoma (POAG). In eyes with XFS and IOP in the statistically normal range, the mean IOP is higher than that in clinically unaffected fellow eyes without XFS. There is a significantly higher IOP and frequency and severity of optic nerve damage at the time of diagnosis, worse visual field damage, poorer response to medications, more severe clinical course, and more frequent necessity for surgical intervention.[9] Glaucomatous damage progresses more rapidly in patients with XFS and glaucoma than in those with POAG. The diurnal fluctuation in IOP is greater in eyes with exfoliative glaucoma than in those with POAG.[10] Glaucoma in XFS is more resistant to medical therapy than is POAG, responds for a shorter period of time, and fails more often.

The IOP in eyes with XFS, with or without medical treatment, tends to fluctuate widely, and in treated eyes in particular, more so than in eyes with POAG. The reason for this can be seen by understanding the pathophysiologic mechanisms underlying the cause of the elevated IOP.[11] Obstruction of the trabecular meshwork either by pigment or XFM or both is generally considered the most likely cause of elevated IOP. The intermediate clear zone is created by rubbing of the iris over the surface of the lens during pupillary movement. With time, these clefts increase in size and begin to become confluent. Eventually, only small bridges may remain as an indication of the previous layer of XFM in the intermediate zone. The liberated exfoliation material is trapped in the trabecular meshwork, which also produced exfoliation material locally.

At the same time, iridolenticular friction leads to disruption of the iris pigment epithelium, resulting in pigment deposition in the trabecular meshwork. Pigment loss from the pupillary ruff and iris sphincter region and its deposition on anterior chamber structures is a hallmark of XFS. This leads to iris sphincter transillumination, loss of the ruff, increased trabecular pigmentation, and pigment deposition on the iris surface. Pigment dispersion in the anterior chamber is common after pupillary dilation and may be profuse. Marked IOP rises can occur after pharmacologic dilation. Post-dilation IOPs should be checked routinely in all patients receiving mydriatics.

Increased trabecular pigmentation is a prominent sign of XFS and may be an early diagnostic finding preceding the appearance of XFM on the pupillary margin or anterior lens capsule.[12] In patients with clinically unilateral involvement, trabecular pigment is almost always denser in the involved eye. Elevated IOP has been correlated with the degree of trabecular pigmentation, and eyes with glaucoma tend to have greater pigmentation than eyes without glaucoma or eyes with POAG.

Glaucomatous damage is usually more advanced in the eye with greater trabecular pigmentation.[13]

Pilocarpine has multiple beneficial actions in eyes with XFS. Not only does it lower IOP, but by increasing aqueous outflow, it should enable the trabecular meshwork to clear more rapidly, and by limiting pupillary movement, should slow the progression of the disease. Aqueous suppressants, on the other hand, by decreasing aqueous secretion, result in decreased aqueous flow through the trabecular meshwork. Becker[14] has presented suggestive evidence that treatment with aqueous suppressants leads to worsening of trabecular function.

The above provides background for addressing two related questions – why does IOP fluctuate more widely in eyes with XFS and why is exfoliative glaucoma harder to control medically? IOP tends to fluctuate more widely in eyes with glaucoma than in ocular hypertensive or normal eyes. Eyes with XFS with or without glaucoma may be prone to IOP spikes resulting from spontaneous liberation of pigment from the iris during pupillary movement or after spontaneous dilation, such as staying for a while in a darkened room. These fluctuations, in turn, may reduce or overcome the IOP lowering effect of antiglaucoma medications, particularly when aqueous suppressants are used.

Drugs which improve aqueous outflow should theoretically be superior to those which reduce aqueous suppression. Miotics have a dual mode of action in eyes with XFS. In addition to increasing trabecular outflow, and perhaps allowing pigment in the meshwork to pass through it, inhibition of pupillary mobility would be expected to reduce or eliminate disruption of the iris pigment epithelium and also eliminate further release of exfoliation material from the lens surface (figure). Theoretically, miotics should be the first line of treatment. However, many patients have nuclear sclerosis and miotics may reduce visual acuity or dim vision sufficiently to create difficulty. We have found that treatment with 2% pilocarpine at bedtime only produces a minimally reactive, non-miotic pupil for 24 hours without interfering with the patient's vision. Prostaglandin analogues, by increasing uveoscleral outflow, in combination with miotics, may provide the best combination of drugs.

In addition, although argon laser trabeculoplasty is highly effective in glaucoma in XFS, approximately 20% of patients develop sudden, late rises of IOP within the first two years after treatment.[15] Continued pigment liberation may overwhelm the restored functional capacity of the trabecular meshwork, and maintenance miotic therapy to minimize papillary movement after laser treatment might counteract this.

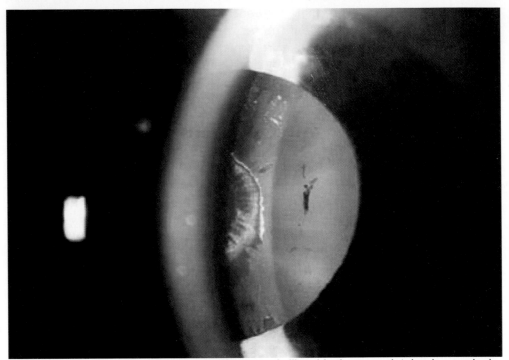

Figure. This patient with exfoliation syndrome and ciliary block was maintained on cycloplegic therapy for over 10 years. The intermediate clear zone has completely filled in. Granular material, similar to that normally present ikn the peripheral zone, is present in both the intermediate zone and central disk, indicating undisturbed buildup of exfoliation material secondary to pupillary immobility.

REFERENCES

1. Ritch R. Exfoliation syndrome: The most common identifiable cause of open-angle glaucoma. J Glaucoma, 1994;3:176-178.

2. Aasved H. Intraocular pressure in eyes with and without fibrillopathia epitheliocapsularis. Acta Ophthalmol, 1971;49:601-610.

3. Kozart DM, Yanoff M. Intraocular pressure status in 100 consecutive patients with exfoliation syndrome. Ophthalmology, 1982;89:214-18.

4. Ringvold A, Blika S, Elsås T. The Middle-Norway eye-screening study. II. Prevalence of simple and capsular glaucoma. Acta Ophthalmol, 1991;69:273-280.

5. Kozobolis VP, Papatzanaki M, Vlachonikolis IG, et al. Epidemiology of pseudoexfoliation in the island of Crete (Greece). Acta Ophthalmol, 1997;75:726-729.

6. Henry JC, Krupin T, Schmitt M, et al. Long-term follow-up of pseudoexfoliation and the development of elevated intraocular pressure. Ophthalmology, 1987;94:545-549.

7. Harju M. Intraocular pressure and progression in exfoliative eyes with ocular hypertension or glauocma. Acta Ophthalmol Scand, 2000;78:699-702.

8. Leske MC, Heijl A, Hussein M, et al. Factors for glaucoma progression and the effect of treatment. The Early Manifest Glaucoma Trial. Arch Ophthalmol, 2003;121:48-56.

9. Konstas AGP, Dimitracoulias N, Konstas PA. Exfoliationssyndrom und Offenwinkelglaukom. Klin Mbl Augenheilkd, 1993;202:259-268.

10. Konstas AGP, Mantziris DA, Stewart WC. Diurnal intraocular pressure in untreated exfoliation and primary open-angle glaucoma. Arch Ophthalmol, 1997;115:182-185.

11. Ritch R, Schlötzer-Schrehardt U, Konstas AGP. Why does glaucoma occur in exfoliation syndrome? Prog Retinal Eye Res, 2003;22:253-275.

12. Prince AM, Streeten BW, Ritch R, et al. Preclinical diagnosis of pseudoexfoliation syndrome. Arch Ophthalmol, 1987;105:1076-1082.

13. Wishart PK, Spaeth GL, Poryzees EM. Anterior chamber angle in the exfoliation syndrome. Br J Ophthalmol, 1985;69:103-105.

14. Becker B. Does hyposecretion of aqueous humor damage the trabecular meshwork? (editorial). J Glaucoma, 1995;4:303-305.

15. Ritch R, Podos SM. Laser trabeculoplasty in exfoliation syndrome. Bull NY Acad Med, 1983;59:339-344.

Question 35

How is neovascular glaucoma most effectively managed?

Shan Lin

Neovascular glaucoma can result from many etiologies and the elevated intraocular pressure is often difficult to control. The final common pathway for the various causes of NVG is the development of a fibrovascular membrane that covers the anterior chamber angle and can cause synechial angle closure.

Retinal ischemia accounts for the vast majority of NVG. It is now being established that neovascular growth in the setting of retinal and/or anterior segment ischemia is mediated by vasoproliferative molecular signals, with the majority of data focused on the role of vascular endothelial growth factor (VEGF).

Treatment of NVG is directed at both eliminating the cause of the neovascularization and reducing the intraocular pressure (IOP). In cases of retinal ischemia, such as central retinal vein or artery occlusion and proliferative diabetic retinopathy, panretinal photocoagulation (PRP) has been shown to be effective in inducing the regression of rubeosis. However, the fibrovascular membrane that covers the angle, and the resultant anterior synechiae that can develop, may not disappear (neovascular vessels become nonpatent but still obstruct the angle), and the IOP remains high. Full PRP should still be performed immediately to halt the progression of the membrane, as well as the angle closure, and to ready the eye for possible surgery which may cause hyphema if the vessels are not functionally closed.

The basis for the medical treatment of NVG is aqueous suppression. Therefore, topical beta-blockers, topical alpha-2 agonists, and topical and systemic carbonic anhydrase inhibitors are the mainstay of therapy.

Prostaglandin analogues may have some efficacy but should be used cautiously. Miotics, including pilocarpine and cholinesterase inhibitors, should be avoided due to their pro-inflammatory effects, miosis, and obstruction of uveoscleral outflow. Atropine is usually recommended for cycloplegia and topical steroids may reduce any accompanying inflammation.

If only a portion of the angle is affected by the fibrovascular membrane and the proliferative process is halted, pharmacological therapy may be sufficient in maintaining a normal IOP. Unfortunately, very often NVG is refractory to medical treatment, and cyclodestructive and/or filtering surgery is necessary. The choice of which specific laser or surgical treatment is most appropriate depends on the severity of the NVG and the visual potential of the eye.

For eyes with relatively good potential vision (e.g., better than hand motions), filtering surgery should be considered the procedure of choice, since the IOP reduction is more predictable and some of the more severe complications associated with cyclophotocoagulation can be avoided.[1]

Both trabeculectomy and tube surgery have been performed with varying efficacy.[1-7] The use of anti-metabolites in trabeculectomy appears to favor successful IOP control in NVG.[2-3] Overall, intra-operative mitomycin-C (MM-C) is more effective than 5-fluorouracil (5-FU) for the control of IOP in refractory glaucomas, but may be associated with a higher rate of Tenons cyst formation.[4]

Tube-shunt procedures have also been shown to be effective in controlling the IOP in cases of NVG.[5-7] Recently, the Ahmed valve has been demonstrated to have relatively good efficacy in NVG series, particularly when used with intra-operative MM-C application.[6-7]

In eyes that have limited or no visual potential, laser cyclophotocoagulation is the preferred surgical therapy. Transscleral cyclophotocoagulation (TCP) is the traditional method for treating the ciliary processes and has good overall results in terms of IOP control.[8] Although easy to perform, TCP has a higher rate of complications such as severe vision loss, hypotony, and IOP failure, when compared to tube-shunt surgery.[1]

Endoscopic cyclophotocoagulation is a novel surgery for the treatment of refractory glaucomas[9-10] and has been successful in limited series of NVG cases.[9-10] This surgical procedure requires an operating room setting and uses an 810-nm diode laser (Endo-Optiks, Little Silver, NJ, USA) with a small handpiece that allows intraocular viewing and treatment of ciliary processes (Fig.1). Since the relative damage to the ciliary region is reduced due to the selective nature of the treatment, the rate of serious complications (hypotony, vision loss) is lower compared to TCP. However, due to its intraocular approach, ECP should be utilized in eyes with some visual potential.

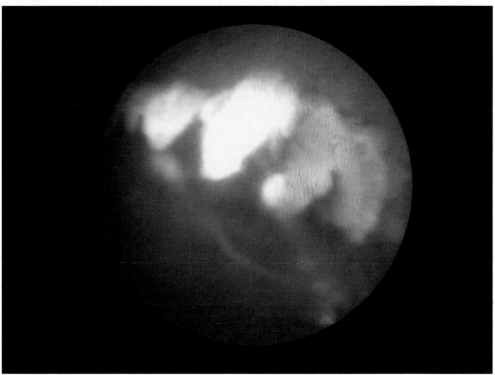

Figure 1. Endoscopic view of ciliary processes treated by endoscopic cyclophotocoagulation (ECP) (white) on the left and illumination of the targeted process by the He-Ne aiming beam immediately to the right.

REFERENCES

1. Eid TE, Katz JL, Spaeth GL, Augsburger JJ. Tube-shunt surgery versus neodymium:YAG cyclophotocoagulation in the management of neovascular glaucoma. Ophthalmology, 1997;104:1692-1700.

2. Mietz H. Risk factors for failures of trabeculectomies performed without antimetabolites. Br J Ophthalmol 1999;83:814-821.

3. Tsai JC, Feuer WJ, Parrish II RK, Grajewski AL. 5-Fluorouracil filtering surgery and neo-vascular glaucoma: long-term follow-up of the original pilot study. Ophthalmology 1995;102:887-893.

4. Katz GJ, Higginbotham EJ, Lichter PR et al. Mitomycin C versus 5-fluorouracil in high-risk glaucoma filtering surgery: extended follow-up. Ophthalmology 1995;102:1263-1269.

5. Mermoud A, Salmon JF, Alexander P, et al. Molteno tube implantation for neovascular glaucoma: long-term results and factors influencing outcome. Ophthalmology 1993;100:897-902.

6. Kook MS, Yoon J, Kim J, Lee MS. Clinical results of Ahmed glaucoma valve implantation in refractory glaucoma with adjunctive mitomycin C. Ophthalmic Surg Lasers. 2000 Mar-Apr;31(2):100-6.

7. Susanna R Jr. Partial Tenon's capsule resection with adjunctive mitomycin C in Ahmed glaucoma valve implant surgery. Br J Ophthalmol. 2003 Aug;87(8):994-8.

8. Bloom PA, Tsai JC, Sharma K, et al. "Cyclodiode": trans-scleral diode laser cyclophoto-coagulation in the treatment of advanced refractory glaucoma. Ophthalmology 1997;104:1508-1520.

9. Chen J, Cohn RA, Lin SC, Cortes AE, Alvarado JA. Endoscopic photocoagulation of the ciliary body for treatment of refractory glaucomas. Am J Ophthalmol. 1997 Dec;124(6):787-96.

10. Uram M. Ophthalmic laser microendoscope ciliary process ablation in the management of neovascular glaucoma. Ophthalmology 1992;99:1823-1828.

Question 36

When is an angle occludable?

S. Fabian Lerner

Closure of the iridocorneal angle by the peripheral iris results in angle closure glaucoma. When the obstruction occurs suddenly, the intraocular pressure rises rapidly, and this condition is called acute angle closure glaucoma (AACG). It is characterized by a sudden, severe and painful onset.

In terms of epidemiology the prevalence of AACG is higher among Eskimos, followed by Asians, Whites and Blacks[1]. Most cases occur in the sixth and seventh decades of life. It is more frequent in females; and in hyperopes, who have smaller eyes and shallower anterior chambers.

AACG occurs in eyes with narrow angles, however not every eye with a narrow angle develops AACG.

Mechanisms of angle closure have been classified by Ritch and Lowe[2] into four groups:

- Pupillary block
- Plateau iris.
- Lens-induced angle closure.
- Malignant (ciliary block) glaucoma.

Pupillary block is the most common cause of angle closure. It may happen as a consequence of posterior synechiae (absolute block), or as a functional block (relative block) which is more frequent.

Gonioscopy is extremely important for an accurate diagnosis and proper treatment. If the patient has a narrow angle, it is important to perform gonioscopy in a dim or dark room with a short beam of light, trying to keep it

167

away from the pupil, as pupillary constriction may make the angle appear deeper.

Different systems for classifying the angle width have been proposed, including the Scheie, the Shaffer, and the Spaeth systems[3]. Shaffer's classification is based on the angular width of the angle recess. In the open angle (20-45°), closure is not possible. In the moderately narrow (20°), or extremely narrow (10°) angle, closure is possible. With a 0° width, the angle is closed. The ophthalmologist should be familiar with one system and write in the chart the structures of the angle that can be seen, the level and angle of iris insertion, pigmentation, and iris contour.

Indentation gonioscopy with a four-mirror type lens should be performed to differentiate appositional from synechial angle closure[4]. After determining the angle configuration, the lens is pressed against the cornea, forcing aqueous to the periphery of the anterior chamber. This pushes the peripheral iris posterior, opening the angle when the closure is appositional, allowing the observer to see deeper structures of the angle. The presence and extension of peripheral anterior synechiae may also be determined with this method. In patients with narrow angles and convex irides (iris bombé), asking the patient to slightly look in the direction of the mirror may allow the examiner to look over the convexity of the iris into the angle.

High frequency ultrasound biomicroscopy (UBM) is a relatively new technique that has helped to understand the mechanisms of angle-closure and measure the angle width[5].

The presence of a narrow angle does not mean that an acute closure will happen. A number of techniques have been used as provocative tests, including the prone test, the dark-room test, and pharmacological dilation of the pupil. Unfortunately due to the high rates of false-positive and false-negative results, the value of these tests in predicting which eyes will develop a spontaneous AACG is uncertain[6].

Treatment with laser peripheral iridotomy (LPI) should be evaluated in the following situations[6,7]:

- Patients with narrow angles and elevated IOP.

- Patients with narrow angles that require pupil dilation or treatment with drugs that may induce pupil dilation.

   – Patients with documented enlargement of the lens provoking progressive closure of the angle.

   – Development of peripheral anterior synechiae.

   – Patients with narrow angle in an only seeing eye.

   – History of limited episodes of halos, blurred vision or pain, characteristic of intermittent and self-limited attacks of angle closure.

   – Inability of rapid evaluation and treatment if an attack develops.

LPI is indicated not only in an eye suffering an AACG but in the fellow eye of patients who have suffered an AACG.

REFERENCES

1. Congdon N, Wang F, Tielsch JM. Issues in the epidemiology and population-based screening of primary angle-closure glaucoma. Survey of Ophthalmology, 36:411-423, 1992.

2. Ritch R, Lowe RF. Angle-closure glaucoma: clinical types. In: Ritch R, Shields MB, Krupin T, editors. The Glaucomas. St. Louis: Mosby, 1996, pp 821-840.

3. Alward WLM. Gonioscopic grading systems. In: Alward WLM: Color Atlas of Gonioscopy. Barcelona: Wolfe, 1994, pp 51-54.

4. Forbes M. Gonioscopy with indentation: a method for distinguishing between appositional closure and synechial closure. Arch Ophthalmol, 1966;76:488-492.

5. Tello C, Tran HV, Liebmann J, Ritch R. Angle closure: classification, concepts, and the role of ultrasound biomicroscopy in diagnosis and treatment. Seminars in Ophthalmology, 2002,17:69-78.

6. Preferred Practice Patterns Committee Glaucoma Panel. Primary Angle-closure glaucoma. Preferred practice pattern. American Academy of Ophthalmology, 1996, pp 6.

7. Hoddap E, Parrish II RK, Anderson DR. Glaucoma suspects III: The abnormal angle. In: Hoddap E, Parrish II RK, Anderson DR. Clinical decisions in glaucoma. St. Louis: Mosby, 1993. pp 148-150.

Question 37

How are occludable angles best detected?
(Management of occludable angles)

Steve K. L. Seah

Tin Aung

Primary angle closure (PACG) is a major form of glaucoma worldwide, particularly in Asia. Recently, a new diagnostic classification of PACG was introduced that focuses on the presence of glaucomatous damage to the optic nerve, as well as damage or obstruction of the trabecular meshwork.[1-2] At the earliest stage of disease, eyes have **occludable angles** without any other abnormality. The term primary angle-closure suspect (PACS) is an alternative term for this condition, as these eyes are at increased risk of developing disease. **Primary angle-closure (PAC)** is said to occur in eyes with synechial angle-closure and/or raised intraocular pressure due to closure of the angle, but without the presence of glaucomatous optic neuropathy. Finally, **primary angle-closure glaucoma (PACG)** is reserved for cases of primary angle-closure with glaucomatous optic neuropathy. Symptomatic or acute angle closure can occur at any stage of this spectrum of disease.

Several epidemiological studies have defined an occludable angle as one in which less than 90° of the posterior pigmented trabecular meshwork is visible on gionioscopy in the primary position of gaze without corneal indentation.[1] Although occludable angles are considered to be the precursors of PAC and PACG, the natural history of the condition is not well established. In a recent population based study, Thomas et al reported that 22% of subjects with PACS develop PAC after 5 years (relative risk 24), but no subject developed PACG.[3] Bilateral PACS was the main risk factor identified for progression to PAC. Although limited by a small sample size with large confidence intervals, this study provided valuable population based prospective data on the natural history and clinical course of occludable angles.

Laser peripheral iridotomy (LPI) is the current standard treatment for angle closure. It acts by alleviating pupillary block present in the condition. In eyes with occludable angles, LPI may halt progression of the angle closure process, and protect against the development of acute symptomatic angle closure. The procedure is safe with few side effects. However it is not established if LPI is necessary for all cases of occludable angles. Performing LPI in all such eyes may not be warranted or cost effective as many eyes would probably never develop progressive disease. Certainly, in countries like China and India with populations exceeding one billion, mass treatment for the large population at risk cannot be recommended at this point of time due to the added burden it will cause to health care providers.

Some eyes with occludable angles may benefit from LPI as they are at greater risk of developing PAC and PACG. An example is the fellow eye of acute angle closure. Such eyes were found to have increased incidence of angle closure,[4-5] and if left untreated, they are at high risk of developing PAC/PACG.[6-7] Prophylactic LPI for fellow eyes has been proven to be beneficial, and studies have demonstrated the effectiveness of iridectomy in preventing acute attacks in fellow eyes.[8,9]

Another factor to be considered in the management of occludable angles is family history. PACG has been found to be more common in first-degree relatives of affected probands than in the general population.[10-13] First-degree relatives of Inuits with PACG were estimated to have a three and a half times greater risk of developing the disorder compared with the general Inuit population.[12] Eyes with occludable angles with a strong family history of PACG may thus benefit from prophylactic LPI treatment. Finally, provocative tests have been used to detect eyes at risk of angle closure.[5,14] Most provocative testing attempts to measure dysfunction using increase in intraocular pressure as the outcome measure. It is likely that prophylactic treatment would also be useful in eyes with occludable angles that have positive provocative tests.

In conclusion, the management of occludable angles requires careful assessment of the eye and patient, with evaluation of the risk of visual loss weighed against the benefit and cost of treatment.

REFERENCES

1. Foster PJ, Johnson GJ. Primary angle-closure-classification and clinical features. In: Hitchings RA, ed. Glaucoma. London: BMJ Publishing Group, 2000.

2. Foster PJ, Buhrmann RR, Quigley HA, Johnson GJ. The definition of glaucoma in prevalence surveys. Br J Ophthalmol, 2002; 86: 238-42.

3. Thomas R, George R, Parikh R, Muliyil J, Jacob A. Five year risk of progression of primary angle closure suspects to primary angle closure: a population based study. Br J Ophthalmol, 2003; 87: 450-4.

4. Sawada A, Sakuma T, Yamamoto T, Kitazawa Y. Appositional angle closure in eyes with narrow angles: comparison between the fellow eyes of acute angle-closure glaucoma and normotensive cases. J Glaucoma 1997; 6: 288-92.

5. Friedman DS, Gazzard G, Foster P, Devereux J, Broman A, Quigley H, Tielsch J, Seah S. Ultrasonographic biomicroscopy, Scheimpflug photography, and novel provocative tests in contralateral eyes of Chinese patients initially seen with acute angle closure. Arch Ophthalmol, 2003; 121: 633-42.

6. Lowe RF. Acute angle-closure glaucoma: the second eye: an analysis of 200 cases. Br J Ophthalmol, 1962; 46: 641-50.

7. Snow JT. Value of prophylactic peripheral iridectomy on the second eye in angle-closure glaucoma. Trans Ophthalmol Soc UK, 1977; 97: 189-91.

8. Fleck BW, Wright E, Fairley EA. A randomized prospective comparison of operative peripheral iridectomy and Nd: YAG laser iridotomy treatment of acute angle closure glaucoma: 3 year visual acuity and intraocular pressure control outcome. Br J Ophthalmol 1997; 81: 884-8.

9. Ang LP. Aung T, Chew PT. Acute primary angle closure in an Asian population: long-term outcome of the fellow eye after prophylactic laser peripheral iridotomy. Ophthalmology, 2000; 107: 2092-6.

10. Lowe RF. Primary angle-closure glaucoma: inheritance and environment. Br J Ophthalmol, 1972; 56: 13-20.

11. Leighton DA. Survey of the first-degree relatives glaucoma patients. Trans Ophthalmol Soc UK 1976; 96: 28-32.

12. Alsbirk PH. Primary angle closure glaucoma: oculometry, epidemiology and genetics in a high-risk population. Acta Ophthalmol (Copenh), 1976; suppl 127: 5-31.

13. Lowe RF. Clinical types of primary angle-closure glaucoma. Aust NZ J Ophthalmol, 1988; 16: 245-50.

14. Lowe RF. Primary angle-closure glaucoma. A review of provocative tests. Br J Ophthalmol 1967; 51: 727-32.

Question 38

Is primary angle-closure glaucoma a single disease?

Robert Ritch

Angle-closure glaucoma consists of several anatomically related conditions in which apposition of the peripheral iris to the functional trabecular meshwork prevents aqueous humor egress from the anterior chamber. These diseases are characterized by abnormalities of the relative or absolute sizes or positions of anterior segment structures and forces which alter the anatomy of the anterior segment in such a way as to cause narrowing of the iridocorneal angle.

The forces causing angle closure may be viewed as originating at four descending anatomic levels: the iris (pupillary block), the ciliary body (plateau iris), the lens (phacomorphic glaucoma), and posterior to the lens (malignant glaucoma).[1] Each level block may also have a component of the mechanisms involved at the preceding levels and may also require the treatment appropriate for each of those levels.

Gonioscopy should always be performed in a completely darkened room using the smallest square of slit-lamp illumination possible (Fig. 1). Indentation gonioscopy is mandatory for accurate differentiation of appositional vs synechial closure.

Pupillary block is an impedance to aqueous flow from the posterior to the anterior chamber through the pupil. Pressure in the posterior chamber is greater than that in the anterior chamber, pushing the peripheral iris forward and narrowing the angle. It may be absolute, as with total posterior synechiae, but most often is functional (relative pupillary block) (Figure 1).

Laser iridotomy is the definitive treatment for angle-closure due to pupillary block.

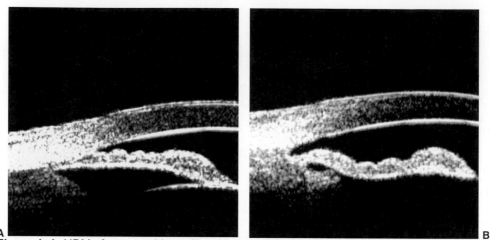

Figure 1. A. UBM of an eye with pupillary block before and after iridotomy. Note that the posterior chamber is large, the ciliary sulcus is prominent, and there is no other structure which could be implicated in causing narrowing of the iridocorneal angle.

Plateau iris configuration refers to an angle appearance in which the iris root angulates forward and then centrally. An anteriorly positioned ciliary body narrows the angle by physically supporting the iris root.[2,3] The iris surface appears flat and the anterior chamber is of relatively normal depth clinically (figure 2). When such an eye develops angle-closure despite a patent iridotomy, it is termed plateau iris syndrome. The level of the iris stroma with respect to the angle structures, or the "height" to which the plateau rises, determines whether or not the angle will close up to the level of Schwalbe's line (complete plateau iris syndrome, in which IOP rises with closure, and is relatively rare) or only partially (incomplete plateau iris syndrome, in which IOP remains normal because the upper meshwork remains open, a far more common situation).[4] Continued appositional angle-closure in the presence of a patent iridotomy is an indication for argon laser peripheral iridoplasty.[5,6]

Anterior lens subluxation or intumescence may precipitate acute angle closure (phacomorphic angle-closure) due to the lens pressing against the iris and ciliary body and forcing them anteriorly. Phacomorphic glaucoma is often unresponsive to medical therapy, and paradoxical reactions to pilocarpine are common and may result in a medically unbreakable attack.[7,8] Peripheral iridoplasty is successful at breaking an acute attack. Iridotomy must be performed within 2-3 days after to eliminate any element of pupillary block, which may also be present.

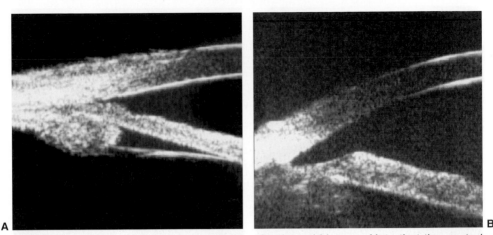

A B

Figure 2. A. UBM of an eye with plateau iris after laser iridotomy. Note that the posterior chamber is extremely small, the ciliary sulcus is nonexistent, and the ciliary processes are prominent and anteriorly positioned, holding the iris against the trabecular meshwork. B. Argon laser peripheral iridoplasty compacts the peripheral iris stroma and opens the angle

Malignant glaucoma (ciliary block) is a multifactorial disease in which increased pressure in the posterior segment causes a pressure differential sufficient to cause forward lens movement and anterior rotation and/or swelling of the ciliary body, leading to direct angle closure by pushing the iris against the trabecular meshwork. Decreased permeability of the anterior hyaloid membrane to fluid transport, zonular laxity, vitreous expansion, and posterior aqueous displacement may play a role in some cases. UBM often reveals a shallow supraciliary detachment not evident on routine B-scan examination. This appears to be the cause of the anterior rotation of the ciliary body and the forward movement of the lens-iris diaphragm.

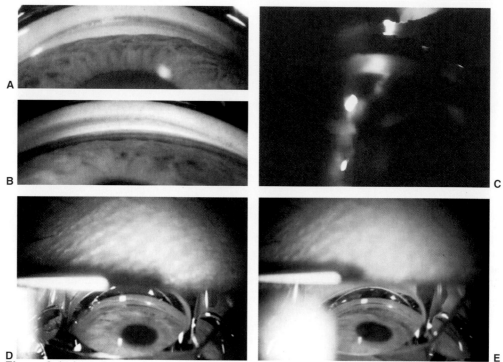

Figure 3. Indentation gonioscopy in pupillary block (upper left), in which the angle opens widely due to the lack of resistance in the distended posterior chamber; plateau iris syndrome (upper right), characterized by the double hump sign, in which the deepest point of indentation is at the periphery of the lens, the beam then rising over the anteriorly placed and large ciliary processes; and 3) lens-induced angle-closure, in which the deepest point of indentation is also at the periphery of the lens but this extends directly into the angle, the iris having a domed appearance as it curves over the anterior lens surface.

REFERENCES

1. Ritch R, Liebmann JM, Tello C. A construct for understanding angle-closure glaucoma: the role of ultrasound biomicroscopy. Ophthalmol Clin N Amer, 1995;8:281-293.

2. Ritch R. Plateau iris is caused by abnormally positioned ciliary processes. J Glaucoma, 1992;1:23-26.

3. Pavlin CJ, Ritch R, Foster FS. Ultrasound biomicroscopy in plateau iris syndrome. Am J Ophthalmol, 1992;113:390-395.

4. Lowe RF, Ritch R. Angle-closure glaucoma: Clinical types. In: Ritch R, Shields MB, Krupin T, ed. The Glaucomas. St. Louis: Mosby, 1989: 839-853. vol 2).

5. Ritch R, Lowe RF, Reyes A. Angle-closure glaucoma - A therapeutic overview. In: Ritch R, Shields MB, Krupin T, ed. The Glaucomas. St. Louis: Mosby, 1989:

6. Ritch R. Argon laser peripheral iridoplasty: an overview. J Glaucoma, 1992;1:206-213.

7. Ritch R. Argon laser treatment for medically unresponsive attacks of angle-closure glaucoma. Am J Ophthalmol, 1982;94:197.

8. Lai JSM, Tham CCY, Chua JKH, Lam DSC. Immediate diode laser peripheral iridoplasty as treatment of acute attack of primary angle-closure glaucoma. A preliminary study. J Glaucoma, 2001;10:89-94.

Question 39

How is acute angle glaucoma managed?

Celso Tello

In acute angle-closure glaucoma there is a rapid elevation of the intraocular pressure due to sudden blockage of the trabecular meshwork by the peripheral iris. The intraocular pressure may rise high enough to cause temporary corneal endothelial cell dysfunction, resulting in_corneal edema. As a result, patients may experience a decrease in visual acuity, halos around lights, intense pain, conjunctival injection, excessive lacrimation and lid edema. In addition, these patients may present with anxiety, fatigue and vasovagal responses such as bradycardia and diaphoresis. On examination, corneal edema may limit the view of the anterior and posterior segments, even after the topical application of glycerin. The anterior chamber may appear moderately shallow and the pupil fixed and mid-dilated. Examination of the fellow eye usually demonstrates a shallow anterior chamber and narrow angle and is useful in differentiating acute angle-closure glaucoma from uveitic, neovascular and phacolytic glaucoma. During the attack, the optic nerve head may be edematous and hyperemic. Spontaneous termination of an acute angle-closure attack can occur as a result of suppression of aqueous secretion caused by the high intraocular pressure or when aqueous from the posterior chamber percolates through areas of newly formed iris atrophy and necrosis, effectively bypassing the pupillary block.

The definitive treatment of acute angle–closure glaucoma is laser iridotomy (LI). Laser iridotomy allows percolation of aqueous humor from the posterior chamber to the anterior chamber, equalizing pressure gradients between these chambers which allows flattening of the peripheral iris and relief of blockage of the trabecular meshwork (Fig. 1A-B).

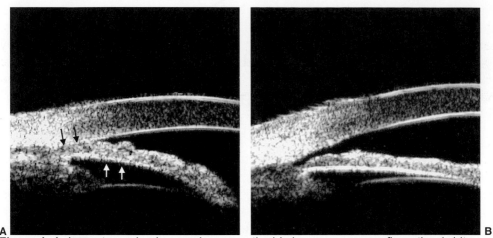

Figure 1. A. In acute angle-closure glaucoma, the iris has a convex configuration (white arrows) due to the relative pressure differential between the posterior chamber and the anterior chamber. The angle is closed (black arrows). B. Following laser iridotomy, aqueous has free access to the anterior chamber and the pressure gradient is eliminated. The iris assumes a flat (planar) configuration and the angle opens.

In clinical practice, patients presenting with an acute angle-closure glaucoma are initially treated with aqueous suppressants including: topical beta blockers, alpha 2 agonists, carbonic anhydrase inhibitors (topical, oral or intravenous) and occasionally hyperosmotics to decrease the intraocular pressure. By decreasing the IOP, the corneal clarity will improve which will facilitate the performance of laser iridotomy. Occasionally, in mild cases, low concentrations of miotics (pilocarpine 2 %) will induce miosis pulling the peripheral iris away from the trabecular meshwork breaking the attack. However, when IOP is quite elevated (above 40-50 mmHg) the pupillary sphincter may be ischemic and unresponsive to miotic agents. Stronger miotics should be avoided since they may increase the vascular congestion of the iris and may rotate the lens-iris diaphragm more anteriorly, worsening the pupillary block.

Several techniques have been described to perform a laser iridotomy, however all surgeons agree that the procedure is performed easily when the attack of glaucoma has been broken either pharmacologically or with indentation gonioscopy. I prefer the "drilling" technique, using the argon laser to photo-coagulate the anterior surface of the iris epithelium and stroma, follow by Nd:YAG-laser. To begin, I use the argon laser (50 microns spot size, 0.02 second duration and 200-300 mW of power) to mark the ideal site for the laser treatment (at 11 o'clock or 1 o'clock position as peripheral as possible under the upper eyelid). Then the settings are adjusted by decreasing the duration to 0.01 second and increasing the power to 800-900 or higher to obtain an adequate response. Once 80 t0 90% of the iris stroma has been photocoagulated I use the Nd-YAG-laser (2.0-3.5 mJ) to penetrate the iris. I find this technique works in all type of irides.

Occasionally, in eyes with hazy-edematous corneas and very shallow anterior chambers, laser iridotomy may be technically difficult. In these cases I use argon laser peripheral iridoplasty (0.5 second duration, 500 microns spot size and low power 200-300 mW) to pull the peripheral iris away from the trabecular meshwork, exposing aqueous humor to the meshwork which may break the attack. By pulling the iris away from the cornea, iridoplasty also facilitates peformance of laser iridotomy.

After the attack has been broken and laser iridotomy performed, the IOP should be controlled medically and steroids should be used to control the inflammation.

REFERENCES

1. Ritch R, Liebmann J, Tello C. A construct for understanding angle-closure glaucoma: the role of ultrasound biomicroscopy. Ophthalmol Clin N Amer, 1995;8:281-93.

2. Ritch R, Shields B, Krupin T. The glaucomas, Clinical Science. St. Louis: Mosby, 1996,821.

3. Liebamnn JM, Ritch R. Laser Iridotomy. Ophthalmic Surgery an Lasers, March, 1996. Vol 27, N3:209-22.

4. Ritch R, Liebamnn J. Argon laser peripheral iridoplasty. Ophthalmic Surgery and Laser, April, 1996. Vol 27,No 4.289-300.

Question 40

How is a patient with chronic angle closure best managed?

Tsing-Hong Wang

Primary chronic angle-closure glaucoma (CACG) refers to a gradual asymptomatic obstruction of the anterior chamber angle by patchy or total peripheral anterior synechiae, and the subsequent rise in intraocular pressure (IOP) and progressive glaucomatous damages that are indistinguishable from that found in chronic open-angle glaucoma. The demographical and anatomical factors play an important role in the development of CACG. The disease is often diagnosed at a late stage and is a major cause of blindness in Asia and could be the most prevalent form of glaucoma in the world[1].

Laser peripheral iridotomy (LPI) is indicated for all stages of CACG[2]. Iridotomy will open those areas of angle not involved by PAS and prevent further synechial closure. However, recent reports found that LPI alone did not prevent most eyes with CACG and glaucomatous damage from developing a clinically significant rise in IOP during extended follow-up[3]. Any persistent or subsequent IOP elevation is treated in a stepwise fashion. First medically, then laser peripheral iridoplasty (gonioplasty) could be used if the angle is still closed. Surgery is indicated in patients who need a lower IOP to preserve their useful visual function.

The need for continued medical treatment after iridectomy is determined by the level of IOP and the extent of glaucomatous damages. Treatment is similar to that of open-angle glaucoma. Prostaglandin analogues were also effective in the treatment of CACG[4].

The need for further surgery can not be predicted from the level of initial IOP or the gonioscopic changes. Iridectomy was indicated for most cases of chronic angle closure without visual filed (VF) loss; however, trabeculectomy might be the best choice in most patients with VF loss and medically uncontrolled pressure. Salmon found that the cup to disk ratio was the best indicator in deciding whether to perform trabeculectomy in eyes that had CACG and had undergone laser iridectomy[5]. The chance of developing malignant glaucoma increases after filtration surgery in patients who have had angle-closure glaucoma.

Removal of the lens may result in an increase in the anterior chamber depth and normalization of IOP in some patients with CACG[6,7]. The choice of first a cataract procedure with the option of a future trabeculectomy may be a more attractive approach in patients with CACG than trabeculectomy followed by an optional cataract procedure[8]. However, the angle may remain closed by the PAS after cataract operation. Goniosynechialysis is a surgical procedure to strip the PAS from the angle wall in an attempt to restore the trabecular function. Additional argon laser peripheral iridoplasty after goniosynechialysis has been used to prevent reclosure of the angle.[9]

The pathophysiology of the angle-closure is not well understood, but various mechanisms or combination of mechanisms may contribute. These mechanisms include relative pupillary block, plateau iris configuration, phacomorphic angle closure, and so on. With the help of new technologies, such as UBM, the classification of CACG is getting more complicated[10]. We also can predict the management principles of CACG will follow this change in the near future.

REFERENCES

1. Congdon N, Wang F, Tielsch JM: Issues in the epidemiology and population-based screening of PACG. Surv Ophthalmol 1992;36:411-23.

2. Robin AL, Pollack IP: Argon laser peripheral iridotomies in the treatment of primary angle-closure glaucoma: long-term follow-up. Arch Ophthalmol 1982;100:919-23.

3. Rosman M, Aung T, Ang LPK et al: Chronic angle-closure with glaucomatous damage – long-term clinical course in a North American population and comparison with an Asian population. Ophthalmology 2002;109:2227-31.

4. Hung PT, Hsieh JW, Chen YF et al: Efficacy of latanoprost as an adjunct to medical therapy for residual angle-closure glaucoma after iridectomy. J Ocul Pharmacol Ther 2000;16:43-7.

5. Salmon JF: Long-term intraocular pressure control after Nd-YAG laser iridectomy in chronic angle-closure glaucoma. J Glaucoma 1993;2:291-6.

6. Gunning FP, Greve EL: Lens extraction for uncontrolled angle-closure glaucoma: Long-term follow-up. J Cataract Refract Surg 1998;24:1347-56.

7. Hayashi K, Hayashi H, Nakao F et al:Changes in anterior chamber angle width and depth after intraocular lens implantation in eyes with glaucoma. Ophthalmology 2000;107:698-703.

8. Greve EL: primary angle-closure glaucoma:extracapsular cataract extraction or filtering procedure? Int Ophthalmol 1988;12:157-62.

9. Lai JSM, Tham CCY, Lam DSC. The efficacy and safety of combined phacoemulsification, intraocular lens implantation, and limited goniosynechialysis, followed by diode laser peripheral iridoplasty, in the treatment of cataract and chronic angle-closure glaucoma. J Glaucoma 2001;10:309-15.

10. Kim YY, Jung HR: Clarifying the nomenclature for primary angle-closure glaucoma. Surv Ophthalmol 1997;42:125-36.

Question 41

How to diagnose and manage glaucoma in nanophthalmic eyes?

Roberto Freire Santiago Malta

Nanophthalmia, or pure microphthalmia, is a rare disease characterized by a significantly reduced ocular globe, a short anterior-posterior axial length, a substantially reduced corneal diameter, besides an anterior chamber with a concave-convex profile and a marked tendency for atalamia and high hypermetropia. This anomaly in ocular development results from an arrest in ocular growth after closure of the orbital fissure. The palpebral fissure is generally narrow and the eye is situated deeply within a small orbit, without there being any systemic abnormality.[1]

Othman et al[2] have carried out a genetic evaluation on a family in which nanophthalmia was transmitted in an autosomal-dominant manner.

Study of the genome revealed that nanophthalmia in this family was the result of a defect in locus NNO1 in Chromosome 11. This same locus has also been detected in a Brazilian family suffering from the disease.[3]

From a biometric standpoint, nanophthalmic eyes present with an average corneal diameter of 10.3 mm, average axial depth in the anterior chamber of 1.46mm, average anterior-posterior axial diameter of 17.00 mm, average crystalline axial thickness of 5.18 mm, a crystalline/eye volume ratio of 12.16% and coroidal-sclera thickness of 2.78mm.[4] In association, these eyes present with corneas which have greatly accentuated curvatures, a closed anterior chamber angle and a highly convex iris.[5]

In conjunction, ultrasound biomicroscopy of nanophthalmic glaucoma affected eyes showed a poor ciliary sulcus with an anterior ciliary body and an iris with a plateau aspect.[6]

Acute glaucoma, malignant glaucoma, uveal effusion, intra-ocular hemorrhaging and nonrhegmatogenous retinal detachment are serious complications which frequently occur in these eyes, both spontaneously and after cataract or glaucoma surgery.

The mechanism of angle closure in nanophthalmic eyes is multifactorial and includes pupillary block, iris appositioning to the sclera wall with possible formation of goniosynechiae and anterior rotation of the ciliary body associated to ciliochoroidal detachment.

Brockhurst et al[7] state that the thickened sclera in these sufferers play a part in the pathogenesis of the uveal effusion, due to the difficulty in draining the fluxo venous through the vortex veins and the reduction in transscleral flow of proteins from the eye. This causes transudation of fluids from the choriocapillaries into the intercellular space.

Studies of the ultrastructure of the sclera in patients with nanophthalmia have shown changes in fiber collagen characteristics through diameter increase and the fraying and disorganization of these.[8]

Practically all nanophthalmic eyes, regardless of having glaucoma or not, must be submitted to iridectomy with YAG laser in order to eliminate the pupillary block component. If, despite iridectomy, apposition of the iris against the trabecular meshwork remains enhanced, peripheral iridoplasty with argon-laser may be considered. Miotics should be used with caution given the paradoxal effect in narrow angles, a result of zonular relaxation with consequent anterior displacement of the crystalline-irido lens.[9]

In cases of uveal effusion or ciliochoroidal detachment, the use of cycloplegics could be beneficial. This medicine relaxes the ciliary muscle, tightening the zonular apparatus and can pull the crystalline lens posteriorly to widen the angle. Occasionally the uveal effusion can be clinically treated with systemic cortisone.

The main surgical complications in nanophthalmic eyes are choroidal detachment, nonregmatogenous retinal detachment, uveal effusion and malignant glaucoma.[7]

Decompression of the vortex veins, anterior sclerotomies and the prophylactic treatment of malignant glaucoma, number some of the procedures which should be used in these patients. In our view, all patients with a classic nanophthalmic pictures, and indicated for cataract and/or glaucoma surgery, should undergo decompression of vortex veins or anterior sclerotomies in the four quadrants at surgery time, in a bid to prevent the above-mentioned complications. In cases of glaucoma with very elevated intra-ocular pressure, the use of hyperosmotic agents, carbonic anhydrase inhibitors, cycloplegics and beta-blockers can occasionally reduce the incidence of malignant glaucoma.[5]

REFERENCES

1. Duke-Elder, S., editor: Anomalies in the size of the eye. In System of Ophthalmology, vol 3, pt 2, St. Louis: Mosby, 1964.

2. Othman, M. I. et al. Autosomal dominant nanophthalmos (NNO1) with high hyperopia and angle-closure glaucoma maps to chromosome11. Am J Hum Genet, 63: 1411-1418, 1998.

3. Malta, R. F. S., Povoa, C. A., Castro, E. F. S., Susanna, R., Giannella-Neto, D. Nanophthalmos (NNO1): Study brazilian family. Arvo Meeting Abstracts, May, 2000; s4370.

4. Singh, O. S., Simmons, R. J., Brockrust, R. J., Trempe, C. L.: Nanophthalmos. A perspective on identification and therapy. Ophthalmology, 89: 1006-1012, 1982.

5. Malta, R. F. S.: Nanoftalmia. Cirurgia de trabeculectomia e descompressão das veias vorticosas associada ao tratamento profilático do glaucoma maligno. Rev Bras Oftal, 52: 69-72, 1993.

6. Barboza, W. L., Malta, R. F. S., Betinjane, A. J.: Nanoftalmia. Aspectos da biomicroscopia ultra-sônica. Arq Bras Oftal, 60: 429, 1997.

7. Brockhurst, R. J.: Vortex vein decompression for nanophthalmia uveal effusion. Arch Opthalmol, 98: 1987-1990, 1980.

8. Stewart III, D. H., Streeten, B. W., Brockhurst, R. J., Anderson, D. R., Hirose, T., Gass, D. M.: Abnormal scleral collagen in nanophthalmos. An ultrastructural study. Arch Ophthalmol, 109: 1017-1025, 1991.

9. Burgoyne, C.: Nanophthalmia and chronic angle-closure glaucoma. J Glaucoma, 11: 525-528, 2002.

Question 42

Which are the limitations of laser iridotomy in the management of primary angle closure glaucoma?

Anita S. Y. Chan

Tin Aung

Paul T. K. Chew

Primary angle closure glaucoma (PACG) is a major cause of visual morbidity in Asia[1]. Epidemiological studies have shown that PACG has high prevalence amongst Asians, especially in populations of Chinese and Mongoloid descent[2-5]. In older people, the incidence of PACG also increases as the lens enlarges and the depth and volume of the anterior chamber decrease.

Recently there has been a shift in the classification of the disease, with an emphasis placed on the presence of glaucomatous damage to the optic nerve as well as the degree of angle obstruction.[6-8] A primary angle closure suspect may have narrow angles without any other abnormality. The definition of narrow angles is based on goniosopic findings. Primary angle closure (PAC) is defined as eyes with narrow angles with peripheral anterior synechiae and/or raised intraocular pressure due to occlusion of the angles but without glaucomatous optic neuropathy. The term PACG is thus reserved for cases with glaucomatous optic neuropathy.

The pathophysiological mechanisms that contribute to PACG include pupillary block as well as non pupil block factors such as lens factors, angle iris crowding and damaged trabecular function.[9-10] However, it has been reported that, pupil block is believed to account for at least 90% of PACG cases in Mongolia.[11]

Laser peripheral iridotomy (LPI) is the current initial treatment in the initial management of PACG. It acts by relieving the pupillary block that is present in the condition.[12-17] LPI has been found to be useful as a prophylaxis against acute attacks of PAC.[18-19] In fellow eyes of acute PAC, prophylactic LPI was found to prevent long-term rise in intraocular pressure (IOP) in 88.8% of fellow eyes after 4 years.[20] However, in affected eyes with acute PAC, a Singapore study found that 58.1% of eyes developed a rise in IOP requiring treatment in spite of the presence of a patent LPI, with the majority of eyes developing a rise in IOP within the first six months of presentation.[21] Almost a third of cases eventually underwent filtering surgery due to uncontrolled IOP, despite laser and medical therapy. These results seem to suggest that LPI alone may not be sufficient as long-term therapy in eyes with acute PAC. Although relatively safe, the use of LPI in angle closure suspects is also not established as the long term clinical course of such eyes is not known. As many eyes would probably not go on to develop the PACG disease, LPI may not be warranted or cost effective in all cases.

Recent studies have highlighted the limitations of LPI in the long term management of PACG. In the early stages of PAC, in the absence of glaucomatous optic nerve damage, LPI has been found to be effective in widening the drainage angle and reducing elevated intraocular pressure.[11] However, in cases of established PACG, LPI was not found to be able to protect against the subsequent rise in intraocular pressure and thus progression of the disease. This is because once extensive synechial angle closure and glaucomatous optic neuropathy have occurred; a patent LPI alone is usually insufficient in controlling the intraocular pressure. Studies in Mongolia have shown that LPI failed in 47% of eyes with PACG.[11] Similarly, in a study in Singapore, as many as 90% of PACG eye treated by LPI needed further medication to control intraocular pressure, with 50% progressing to require filtering surgery.[23] Most of those who developed a rise in IOP after LPI were found to do so within the first 6 months. The same study methodology used in a study in New York of Caucasian subjects also confirmed the limitations of LPI in established PACG.[22] In that study, most eyes needed further treatment to control the intraocular pressure, with medical therapy failing in at least a third of the cases, necessitating further laser treatment or filtering surgery. These results in Asian and American populations indicate that the limitations of LPI in the management of PACG are not related to racial or ethnic variation.

Long term management of PACG eyes treated with LPI therefore consists of monitoring for cases that develop inadequate control of intraocular pressure and controlling any persistent or subsequent rise in intraocular pressure in a stepwise fashion, with medications first and subsequently, laser or surgery. Surgical options include filtering surgery, lens extraction, angle-widening procedures or a combination of these procedures.

In conclusion, although LPI is useful in relieving the initial mechanism of pupillary block in angle closure, it cannot be relied on for the long term control of the intraocular pressure. Once synechial closure and optic nerve damage has occurred, other treatment options would have to be used in combination in order to adequately control the intraocular pressure. This has significant implications for developing countries in Asia with high prevalence of PACG.

If PACG patients are not followed up closely after LPI, they risk suffering further glaucomatous visual damage and blindness.

REFERENCES

1. Quigley HA, Congdon NG, Friedman DG. Glaucoma in China (and worldwide): changes in established thinking will decrease preventable blindness. Br J Ophthalmol, 2001; 85:1271-1272.

2. Foster PJ, Baasanhu J, Alsbirk P, et al. Glaucoma in Mongolia- a population based survey in Hovsgol Province, Northern Mongolia. Arch Ophthalmol, 1996; 114: 1235-41.

3. Foster PJ, Oen FT, Machin D, et al. The prevalence of glaucoma in Chinese residents of Singapore: a cross-sectional population survey of the Tanjong Pagar district. Arch Ophthalmol, 2000;118: 1105-11.

4. Dandona L, Dandona R, Mandal P, et al. Angle closure glaucoma in an urban population in Southern India. The Andhra Pradesh Eye Disease Study. Ophthalmology, 2000; 107: 1710-6.

5. Foster PJ, Johnson GJ. Glaucoma in China: how big is the problem? Br J Ophthalmol, 2001;85:1277-82.

6. Devereux JG, Foster PJ, Baasanhu J, et al. Anterior chamber depth measurement as a screening toll for primary angle losure glaucoma in an East Asian population. Arch Ophthalmol, 2000; 118: 257-63.

7. Foster PJ, Johnson GJ. Primary angle-closure-classification and clinical features. In: Hitchings RA, ed. Glaucoma. London: BMJ Publishing Group, 2000. A summary of the new nomenclature used in PACG.

8. Foster PJ, Buhrmann RR, Quigley HA, et al. The definition of glaucoma in prevalence surveys. Br J Ophthalmol, 2002; 86: 238-42

9. Hung PT, Chou LH. Provocation and mechanism of angle-closure glaucoma after iridectomy. Arch Ophthalmol, 1979; 97:1862-4.

10. Ritch R, Lowe RF, Reyes A: Therapeutic overview of angle-closure glaucoma, in Ritch R, Shields MB, Krupin T (eds): The Glaucomas, St Louis: Mosby, 1989, pp 855-864.

11. Nolan WP, Foster PJ, Devereux JG, Uranchimeg D, Johnson GJ, Baasanhu J. YAG laser iridotomy treatment for primary angle-closure in East Asian eyes. Br J Ophthalmol, 2000; 84:1255-1259.

12. Ritch R. The treatment of chronic angle-closure glaucoma. Ann Ophthalmol, 1981; 13:21-3.

13. Robin AL, Pollack IP. Argon laser peripheral iridotomies in the treatment of primary angle-closure glaucoma: long term follow-up. Arch Ophthalmol, 1982;100:919-23.

14. Quigley HA. Long-term follow-up of laser iridotomy. Ophthalmology, 1981;88:218-24.

15. Gieser DK, Wilensky JT. Laser iridectomy in the management of chronic angle-closure glaucoma. Am J Ophthalmol, 1984;98:446-50.

16. Schwartz LW, Moster MR, Spaeth GL, et al. Neodynium-YAG laser iridectomies in glaucoma associated with closed or occludeable angles. Am J Ophthalmol, 1986;102:41-4.

17. Salmon JF. Long-term intraocular pressure control after Nd-YAG laser iridotomy in chronic angle-closure glaucoma. J Glaucoma, 1993;2:291-6.

18. Wilensky JT. Narrow angles accompanied by slit-lamp and gonioscopic evidence of risk are indications for prophylactic laser iridectomy. Surv Ophthalmol, 1996; 41: 31-2.

19. Ritch R. Definitive signs and gonioscopic visualization of appositional angle closure are indications for prophylactic laser iridectomy. Surv Ophthalmol, 1996; 41: 33-6.

20. Ang LP. Aung T, Chew PT. Acute primary angle closure in an Asian population: long-term outcome of the fellow eye after prophylactic laser peripheral iridotomy. Ophthalmology, 2000;107:2092-6.

21. Aung T, Ang LP, Chan SP, Chew PT. Acute primary angle-closure: long-term intraocular pressure outcome in Asian eyes. Am J Ophthalmol, 2001;131: 7-12.

22. Alsagoff Z, Aung T, Ang LPK, Chew PTK. Long-term clinical course of primary angle-closure glaucoma in an Asian population. Ophthalmology, 2000; 107: 2300-2304.

23. Rosman M, Aung T, Ang LPK, Chew PTK, Liebmann J, Ritch R. Chronic Angle-Closure with Glaucomatous Damage: Long-term Clinical Course in a North American population and comparison with an Asian Population. Ophthalmology, 2002; 109: 2227-31.

Question 43

How is malignant glaucoma diagnosed and treated?

Jody Piltz-Seymour

Malignant glaucoma, also known as ciliary block glaucoma, is a relatively uncommon form of secondary glaucoma[1,2]. It is caused when the aqueous is blocked from moving towards the anterior chamber and becomes trapped posteriorly in the vitreous cavity. The increasing volume of aqueous in or behind the vitreous causes expansion of the vitreous cavity, flattening of the anterior chamber and elevation of the intraocular pressure. The alternate names for malignant glaucoma refer to the theory that the ciliary processes "block" the forward movement of aqueous by adhering to the lens equator or anterior hyaloid face causing aqueous to be "misdirected" posteriorly. As the vitreous gel is pushed forward, the anterior hyaloid becomes compacted impairing its permeability.

How is malignant glaucoma diagnosed?

The diagnosis of malignant glaucoma depends on recognizing key clinical features, particularly in high risk patients[3]. Malignant glaucoma presents with shallowing, often with complete flattening, of the anterior chamber associated with elevated intraocular pressure. The lens, intraocular lens or hyaloid is often pressed against the corneal endothelium. Patients present with pain, which may be severe, red eye, corneal edema, and decreased vision. Other symptoms associated with elevated IOP may be present, such as headache, nausea, and vomiting.

Malignant glaucoma develops most commonly after glaucoma surgery in eyes with prior angle closure, but it can develop after any intraocular surgery or laser, upon initiating miotic therapy and, rarely, it can develop spontaneously. Ultrasound biomicroscopy can help confirm the diagnosis [4].

Malignant glaucoma needs to be differentiated from pupil block and suprachoroidal hemorrhage, both of which can present with shallow anterior chamber and elevated intraocular pressure. The eyes with pupil block have shallow peripheral anterior chambers with iris bombe, but the central chamber does not completely flatten. A patent iridotomy is usually required to rule out pupil block. The diagnosis of suprachoroidal hemorrhage is usually apparent on fundus examination and/or ultrasound evaluation.

How is malignant glaucoma treated?

Aggressive medical therapy should be instituted as soon as malignant glaucoma is suspected in an eye with a patent iridotomy [2,5]. Cycloplegia helps tighten the zonules, pulling the lens-iris diaphram posteriorly, which helps to break the ciliary block. Cycloplegia with atropine 1% is often combined with a mydriatic, typically phenylephrine 2.5% or 10%. Topical β-blockers and topical or systemic carbonic anhydrase inhibitors are useful in diminishing aqueous production. Hyperosmotic agents, such as glycerol or mannitol, lower intraocular pressure and dehydrate the vitreous; they help expand the anterior chamber, allow the lens-iris diaphram to move posteriorly and de-compact the anterior hyaloid membrane. Miotics are contraindicated, as they cause forward movement of the lens-iris diaphram and worsening of the ciliary block.

Medication is usually effective in breaking the ciliary block in 50% of cases. Long term or permanent use of cycloplegia may be required to prevent reoccurrences. If up to 5 days of medical therapy is unsuccessful, laser and/or surgical therapy should be instituted [5,6]. Yag laser lysis of the posterior capsule and anterior hyaloid membrane has been shown to break the malignant glaucoma in pseudophakes in numerous reports, but results may sometimes be transient. Others have advocated argon laser treatment to shrink ciliary processes visible through an iridectomy. While Chandler's procedure of tapping the vitreous using an 18guage needle through a posterior sclerotomy can be effective, mechanical pars plana vitrectomy is preferable if available. It is imperative to remove the anterior hyaloid membrane. It is also vital to ensure that there is a sizable communication into the anterior chamber, as inflammation from the malignant glaucoma may compromise the patency of a small iridectomy. Also, if the precipitating surgery was a trabeculectomy, it is important to try to re-establish filtration intraoperatively.

Unfortunately, despite aggressive medical and surgical treatment, the disease can occasionally take a 'malignant' course with the development of fibrosis in the anterior segment postoperatively, resulting in redevelopment of block, often with ciliary and pupillary block components[7,8]. These rare, post-vitrectomized eyes may respond to removal of the IOL or pars plana insertion of a glaucoma drainage device.

Fellow eyes of affected patients are predisposed to developing malignant glaucoma. Miotics should be avoided. Consideration should be given to performing an iridotomy before intraocular surgery and administering cycloplegia after intraocular surgery.

REFERENCES

1. Simmons RJ: Malignant glaucoma. Br J Ophthalmol, 56:273, 1972.

2. Simmons RJ, Maestre FA: Malignant glaucoma. In Ritch R, Shields MB, Krupin T eds. The Glaucomas, St. Louis: Mosby, 1996 pp 841-855.

3. Trope G, et al: Malignant glaucoma: clinical and ultrasound biomicrocopic characteristics. Ophthlamology, 101:1030, 1994.

4. Tello C, Chi T, Shepps G, et al. Ultrasound biomicrosopy in pseudophakic malignant glaucoma. Ophthalmology, 100: 1330-1334, 1993.

5. Chandler PA, Simmons RJ, GrantWM: Malignant glaucoma: medical and surgical treatment. Am J Ophthalmol, 66:495-502, 1968

6. Tsai JC, Barton KA, Miller MH, et al. Surgical results in malignant glaucoma refractory to medical or laser therapy. Eye, 11:677-681, 1997.

7. Massicotte E, Schuman JS: A malignant glaucoma-like syndrome following pars plana vitrectomy. Ophthalmology, 106:1375-1379, 1999.

8. Zacharia PT, Abboud EB. Recalcitrant malignant glaucoma following pars plana vitrectomy, scleral buckle, and extracapsular cataract extraction with posterior chamber intraocular lens implantation. Ophthalmic Surg Lasers, 29:323-327, 1998.

Question 44

When should we do laser trabeculoplasty in the management of glaucoma?

Clive Migdal

Laser trabeculoplasty (LTP) is a simple and cost-effective method of reducing intraocular pressure (IOP) in patients with open angle glaucoma. Initial enthusiasm and promise has been followed by results of clinical trials, providing evidence of both short- and long-term effectiveness, and suggesting a specific place for laser therapy in individually selected patients.

Argon laser trabeculoplasty (ALT) was introduced as a treatment option in 1979 following a report by Wise and Witter[1] who presented a method of argon laser photocoagulation of the trabecular meshwork (TM) in phakic open angle glaucoma eyes that had failed medical therapy. The importance of using short-duration (0.1 second) laser applications was emphasized.

Mechanism

This treatment reduces outflow resistance by causing minute, localized burns of the TM, without perforation. The exact mechanism of the effect on the TM, whether mechanical or biochemical, is still not resolved. It has been speculated that healing after circumferential treatment caused contraction of the burn sites, with resultant stretching of the untreated trabeculum, pulling open adjacent intertrabecular spaces. Other hypotheses include that a biochemical response to laser-induced cellular injury accounts for improved outflow[2].

Method

The angle structures are viewed through a goniolens after the instillation of a topical anaesthetic. Laser burns are placed between the anterior pigmented TM and the non-pigmented TM. If burns are placed too posteriorly, they will result in peripheral anterior synechiae (PAS) formation. For this reason, patients with narrow drainage angles are not suitable for LTP as they tend to form PAS.

The amount of laser delivered to the TM is a function of power, duration and spot size. Suggested settings are: spot size 50 microns, duration 0.1 seconds, and power 500 - 1200 mW.

The power is adjusted in order to cause minimal blanching or minute gas bubble formation. The reaction seen will depend on the amount of pigment in the TM. Excesive power should not be used as this may result in unnecessary scarring and subsequent increase in the IOP. In most instances approximately 50 burns are applied to each half of the circumference of the TM. Treatment is usually performed in two separate sessions, separated by a period of two weeks. Some physicians only treat the second half of the angle if the initial treatment does not adequately lower the IOP, or if the IOP increases again at a later date.

To prevent a post-operative treatment spike, the patient can be treated with apraclonidine 1% instilled immediately before or after the laser. The IOP should be checked approximately 30 to 60 minutes post-laser.

Indications

ALT may be considered for patients with POAG, pigmentary glaucoma or pseudoexfoliation glaucoma when the IOP is inadequately controlled with medical therapy (usually up to two topical medications). In selected patients, such as the elderly with poor compliance , or the inability to use drops, ALT may be used as initial therapy.

LTP is contraindicated in patients with uveitic, angle-recession, rubeotic and infantile and juvenile-onset glaucomas. The IOP reduction is usually smaller and short-lived, and considerable increase may occur in retreatment, which is generally avoided.

Complications

The commonest complication is a transient rise in IOP within the first six hours after treatment. This may be minimized by treating only half the angle at one sitting, and by using Apraclonidine 1% in conjunction with the treatment.[3]

Mild iritis is also seen after LTP. Gutt Predsol 0.5% q.i.d. is prescribed for 5 days after laser to reduce this.

A sudden sustained rise in IOP may occur some time after ALT in some patients, probably due to scarring of the TM. For this reason, it is important to maintain regular routine long-term follow-up.

Efficacy

ALT reduces IOP in approximately 85% of treated eyes, with the hypotensive effect usually evident within four weeks of treatment. Studies have shown an initial reduction in the IOP of approximately 20-30% (6-9 mmHg)[4,5]. Patients in the Glaucoma Laser Trial achieved a mean reduction in IOP of 9 mmHg[5]. Large reductions in IOP may also be seen in patients with pseudoexfoliation or pigmentary glaucomas. Aphakic eyes respond less well than phakic ones[4].

It may be possible to reduce or stop adjunctive medication after ALT, thus improving the quality of life of the patient. However, several studies have shown a diminished IOP effect with time, so that by 10 years, more than half the treated eyes required further surgery.

Although ALT is simple to perform, the effect of this treatment on intraocular pressure (IOP) decreases over time in many patients[6]. This fact needs to be considered when assessing an individual for treatment. Other studies, however, have shown an encouraging long-term effect[7,8], with increased outflow facility and a delay in needing to perform trabeculectomy. There were few serious early or late complications. It is important to treat only eyes with open angles, as narrow angles tend to predispose to post-treatment peripheral anterior synechiae, with a subsequent rise in IOP. Less successful outcomes are obtained in aphakic eyes, congenital, juvenile-onset, uveitic or traumatic glaucomas.

Other than Argon, other forms of laser trabeculoplasty have been tried and found effective, such as the diode laser (continuous wave laser of red and infrared wavelengths)[9], and the YAG (532nm) laser (large spot size, high power, low energy, Q-switched, frequency doubled system - also known as Selective Laser Trabeculoplasty)[10]. The latter pulsed system induces minimal scarring, supporting the biochemical hypothesis to explain the laser effect of successfully reducing IOP.

Repeating the argon laser trabeculoplasty if the IOP increases frequently results in substantial increases in IOP[11] with the result that this is now contraindicated. It has, however, been suggested that Selective Laser Trabeculoplasty can be successfully repeated[10], although there are no long-term clinical trials to support this.

Clinical trials

The early published clinical studies showed that most eyes still required adjunctive medical therapy in order to control the IOP. They also showed that, with time, IOPs tended to rise again in many patients, with these requiring further therapy[7].

A number of clinical trials have been designed to investigate LTP as the initial treatment for glaucoma, compared with other treatments such as medicines or surgery. The Moorfields Primary Therapy Trial (commenced in 1983) compared long-term outcomes after random assignment of newly diagnosed mainly Caucasian glaucoma patients to treatment with either laser, medicine or surgery[12]. It was found that medicines and laser (the latter allowed adjunctive pilocarpine where the IOPs were not adequately reduced by laser alone) lowered the IOP to a similar degree. In this study, the group treated with initial surgery showed better IOP-lowering and field preservation than the laser or medical groups.

The Glaucoma Laser Trial (GLT) randomly assigned newly diagnosed patients to either medications or argon LTP. The fellow eye received the opposite treatment from the trial eye [5,13,14]. This study showed a lasting effect of LTP on lowering IOP and preserving visual fields, at least as well as medical treatment. In addition, the laser treated eyes required fewer medications over the duration of the studies[14].

The Advanced Glaucoma Intervention Study (AGIS) tested the effect of two different sequences of treatment on the preservation of visual field if initial medical treatment had failed, namely either ALT followed by trabeculectomy if the laser failed, followed by a repeat trabeculectomy if the first one failed, or trabeculectomy followed by ALT followed by trabeculectomy. A target pressure of 18 mmHg was set for the study, and all interventions were supplemented with medical treatment, if required, to maintain the IOP below 18mmHg. After 5 years of follow-up there was little difference in outcome between the groups. However, an analysis of risk factors indicated that black race increased the risk of failure of IOP control and visual field deterioration after initial trabeculectomy compared with whites after initial trabeculoplasty. Blacks had better outcomes with the sequence starting with trabeculoplasty[15]. In contrast, white patients had approximately equal outcomes from the two treatment sequences for the first two years, after which there was a clear advantage of the sequence starting with trabeculectomy. Data suggested that trabeculoplasty as initial treatment after medication failure slowed progression of field defects more in black than in white patients[15].

From these studies, it can be estimated that, for newly diagnosed primary open angle glaucoma patients, trabeculoplasty may be at least as effective at preserving visual field as medications in some patients for a reasonable period of time (sometimes up to 7 years). For those who have not been controlled after starting medical treatment, black patients have better field preservation than whites if the subsequent treatment chosen is laser (whites do better with trabeculectomy).

Conclusion

LTP (whether performed with blue, green, red or infrared energy), and selective LTP, reduce IOP, although adjunctive medications are frequently required to ensure adequate IOP reduction after this procedure. Post-laser pressure spikes may be smaller or avoided altogether if treatment is performed in two 180 degree steps (although one 180 treatment may also be sufficient to control the IOP in some cases).

Laser trabeculoplasty can be considered as an alternative to medications as initial therapy for some patients, particularly the elderly, infirm and those patients who have a short life expectancy. As second line treatment where medical treatment has failed, LTP has better results in black patients.

Although ALT is simple to perform and cost-effective, the question of long-term IOP control by this procedure remains and patients do need to be monitored continuously as IOP control can be suddenly lost. The ophthalmologist carrying out ALT must have a good knowledge of the anatomy of the drainage angle and be competent at gonioscopy.

REFERENCES

1. Wise JB, Witter SL. Argon laser therapy for open angle glaucoma. A pilot study. Arch Ophthalmol, 1979; 97: 319-322.

2. Van Buskirk EM, Pond V, Rosenquist RC, Acott TS. Argon laser trabeculoplasty. Studies of mechanism of action. Ophthalmology, 1984; 91: 1005-1010.

3. Robin AL. The role of apraclonidine hydrochloride in laser therapy for glaucoma. Trans Am Ophthalmol Soc, 1989; 87: 729-761.

4. Shingleton BJ, Richter CV, Bellows AR, et al. Long-term efficacy of argon laser trabeculoplasty. Ophthalmology, 1987; 94: 1513-1528.

5. Glaucoma Laser trial Research Group. The Glaucoma Laser Trial (GLT): 2. Results of argon laser trabeculoplasty versus topical medicines. Ophthalomology, 1990; 97: 1403-1414.

6. Weinreb RN, Ruderman J, Justen R, et al. Immediate intraocular pressure response to argon laser trabeculoplasty. Am J Ophthalmol, 1983; 95: 279-286.

7. Schwartz Al, Love DC, Schwartz MA. Long-term follow-up of argon alser trabeculoplasty for uncontrolled open angle glaucoma. Arch Ophthalmol, 1985; 103: 1482-4.

8. Wise JB. Ten year results of laser trabeculoplasty. Does laser avoid glaucoma surgery or merely defer it? Eye, 1987; 1: 45-50.

9. Moriarty AP, McHugh JDA, ffytche TJ, Marshall J, Hamilton AMP. Long-term follow-up of diode laser trabeculoplasty for primary open angle glaucoma and ocular hypertension. Ophthalmology, 1993; 100: 1614-1618.

10. Lattina MA, Sibayan SA, Shin DH, Noecker RJ, Marcellino G. Q-switched 532nm Nd:YAG laser trabeculoplasty (selective laser trabeculoplasty). A multicenter pilot clinical study. Ophthalmology, 1998; 105: 2082-2090.

11. Richter CU, Shingleton BJ,Bellows AR, Hutchinson BT, Jacobson LP. Retreatment with argon laser trabeculoplasty. Ophthalmology, 1987; 94: 1085-1089.

12. Migdal C, Gregory W, Hitchings R. Long-term functional outcome after early surgery compared with laser and medicine in open angle glaucoma. Ophthalmology, 1994; 101: 1651-1656.

13. Glaucoma Laser Trial Research Group. The Glaucoma Laser Trial (GLT): 6. Treatment group differences in visual field changes. Am J Ophthalmol, 1995; 120: 10-22.

14. Glaucoma Laser Trial Research Group. The Glaucoma Laser Trial (GLT) and glaucoma laser trial follow up study: 7. Results. Am J Ophthalmol, 1995; 120:718-731.

15. The AGIS Investigators. The Advanced Glaucoma Intervention Study (AGIS): 4. Comparison of treatment outcomes within race. Seven-year results. Ophthalmology, 1998; 105: 1146-1164.

16. The AGIS Investigators. The Advanced Glaucoma Intervention Study (AGIS): 9. Comparison of glaucoma outcomes in black and white patients within treatment groups. Am J Ophthalmol, 2001; 132: 311-320.

Question 45

Is there a role for selective laser trabeculoplasty?

Karim F. Damji

Introduction

Although medical therapy is often utilized as an initial management strategy to lower intraocular pressure (IOP) in glaucoma patients, laser trabeculoplasty may offer a cost-effective alternative.[1] One laser treatment can have a sustained pressure lowering effect for years, which can avoid problems with patient compliance. With a safety and efficacy profile similar to ALT for IOP reduction, as well as its preservation of meshwork architecture and ease of use, SLT is a reasonable alternative to ALT for most glaucoma patients.[2] In addition, far less coagulative damage to the TM, may make it a repeatable procedure.

Background

In primary open-angle glaucoma (POAG), Argon Laser Trabeculoplasty (ALT) has been found to be effective in reducing outflow resistance and permitting increased aqueous outflow through the trabecular meshwork (TM).[3] Recently, a novel, Q-switched, frequency-doubled Nd:YAG laser (532 nm) has been described for use in trabeculoplasty,[4-6] and has been termed Selective Laser Trabeculoplasty (SLT). In tissue culture, it has been demonstrated that the low power and short duration of this laser can selectively target pigmented trabecular meshwork cells, while sparing adjacent cells and tissues from collateral thermal damage, leaving the TM architecture intact.[5,7]

Selectivity

Selective TM targeting relies on a principle known as "selective photothermolysis," which ensures that heat diffusion is confined to the irradiated cell with minimal or no collateral damage.[8] This is achieved by the pulse duration of the laser being shorter that the thermal relaxation time of the target chromophore, which is melanin within pigmented TM cells. A study by Kramer and Noecker using transmission electron microscopy found no TM architectural change in SLT-treated eyes, either in animal models or in human eyes[9] This may be important for patients who require repeat laser treatments or for future surgical therapies where an unaltered TM is beneficial.

IOP lowering with SLT and comparison to ALT

Latina et al.[6] demonstrated safety and efficacy of SLT in an uncontrolled multi-center pilot study. We performed a prospective randomized study in 165 eyes with open-angle glaucoma (including pigmentary and pseudoexfoliation glaucoma) comparing SLT to ALT (results were presented at the International Glaucoma Society meeting in Barcelona, March 21, 2003). We found that at 6 months, 1, 2, and 3 years there was no statistically significant difference in the IOPs of eyes treated with SLT versus those treated with ALT (Table 1). The number of medications used at each visit was comparable in the two groups.

The adverse reactions in each group, including IOP spikes at one hour, number of eyes that went on to have repeat laser and/or surgical interventions, as well as number of eyes requiring additional medication, laser, or surgery for IOP control, was similar in both groups.

We conclude that there is no difference in the IOP lowering effect between SLT and ALT at various time points up to 3 years after initial treatment.

More recently, Melamed et al. have demonstrated that SLT can be used to lower IOP by about 30% in patients with ocular hypertension or those with newly diagnosed primary open-angle glaucoma.[10]

Table 1. Tips for SLT patient selection

Patients for whom SLT is suggested

- Primary open-angle glaucoma, pseudoexfoliation glaucoma or pigmentary glaucoma with medically uncontrolled IOP
- Possibly as first line in those with ocular hypertension or primary open-angle glaucoma (pending further evidence)
- Other secondary open-angle glaucomas
- Previous "failed" argon laser trabeculoplasty (ALT)
- Patients in whom compliance is questionable
- Patients who cannot afford medications
- Patients who wish to reduce the number of medications they are taking
- Patients intolerant of drop therapy

Patients not likely to be good candidates for SLT

- History of or active uveitis
- Neovascular glaucoma
- Traumatic glaucoma
- Congenital or early childhood glaucoma
- Primary or secondary angle-closure glaucoma
- Inadequate visualization of the trabecular meshwork (if pupillary block is present, consider peripheral iridotomy first)

Suggested indications for SLT

Current indications and relative contraindications for treatment with SLT are listed in Table I.

Because of the non-destructive and potentially repeatable properties of SLT, it is attractive to consider this treatment modality as a first-line therapy for open-angle glaucoma and glaucoma suspects.[10] However, a randomized trial comparing SLT to medical therapy in patients with early open-angle glaucoma has not yet been reported.

Treatment settings for SLT are discussed in depth in a recent review.[2] It is worth restating, however, that in cases of pigmentary glaucoma, much lower energy settings should be used (probably around 0.4-0.6mj/pulse) in order to avoid decompensation of a partially damaged TM (this is especially important in advanced pigmentary glaucoma).

Conclusions

Selective laser trabeculoplasty appears to be a safe and effective therapy for lowering intraocular pressure in patients with open-angle glaucoma. It may also be useful for first line therapy in patients with glaucoma or glaucoma suspects, although this awaits further study, as does the potential repeatability of the laser. As we gain more experience, SLT has the potential to supplant ALT for laser trabeculoplasty.

REFERENCES

1. The Glaucoma Laser Trial Research Group: The Glaucoma Laser Trial (GLT), II: Results of argon laser trabeculoplasty vs topical medicines. Ophthalmology, 1990; 97: 1403-1413.

2. Damji KF, Bovell AM, Hodge WG. Selective laser trabeculoplasty. A review and comparison to Argon Laser Trabeculoplasty. Ophthalmic Practice, 2003;21:54-58.

3. Wise JB, Witter SL. Argon laser therapy for open-angle glaucoma: a pilot study. Arch Ophthalmol, 1979; 97: 319-328.

4. Mermound A, Herbort CP, Schnyder CC, et al. Comparison of the effects of trabeculoplasty using the Nd:YAG laser and argon laser. Klin Monatsbl Augenheilkd, 1992; 200: 404-406.

5. Latina MA, Park C. Selective targeting of trabecular meshwork cells: in vitro studies of pulsed and cw laser interactions. Exp Eye Res, 1995; 60: 359-372.

6. Latina MA, Sibayan SA, Shin DH, et al. Q-switched 532-nm Nd:YAG laser trabeculoplasty (selective laser trabeculoplasty): a multicenter, pilot, clinical study. Ophthalmology, 1998; 105: 2082-2090.

7. Hollo G. Argon and low energy pulsed Nd:YAG laser trabeculoplasty. A prospective, comparative clinical and morphological study. Acta Ophthalmol Scand, 1996; 74: 126-131.

8. Anderson RR, Parrish JA. Selective photothermolysis: precise microsurgery by selective absorption of pulsed radiation. Science, New series, April, 29, 1983; 220(4596): 524-527.

9. Kramer TR, Noecker RJ. Comparison of the morphological changes after selective laser trabeculoplasty in human eye bank eyes. Ophthalmology, 2001; 108: 773-779.

10. Melamed S, Ben Simon GJ, Levkovitch-Verin H. Selective Laser Trabeculoplasty as Primary Treatment of Open-angle Glaucoma: A prospective, non-randomized pilot study. Arch Ophthalmol, 2003;121:957-960.

Question 46

When should a laser iridoplasty be performed?

Curt Hartleben

Argon laser peripheral iridoplasty (ALPI), sometimes also caller laser gonioplasty, is used to mechanically open the appositionally closed angle in Primary Angle Closure Glaucoma (PACG). It is most useful when a yag laser iridotomy cannot be performed because of a very narrow angle and flat chamber, where the corneal endothelium or stroma can be damaged by reflected energy, causing mild to severe thermal burns. In other cases, when there is substantial corneal edema, a laser iridotomy is not possible due to lack of visualization of the iris structures. In some cases, it is helpful in refractory cases to help break an acute attack. It can be useful in some narrow-angle glaucomas with mechanisms different than papillary block, such as iris plateau syndrome, iridocilary cysts or nanophthtalmos.[1-4]

Currently, it is most frequently used as an ancillary procedure added to a yag laser iridotomy in PACG where significant narrowing exists after the iridotomy. It is also used with some frequency to lower IOP in patients with acute PACG in refractory cases, especially where there is a mid-dilated pupil or significant corneal haze, which impede a yag laser iridotomy. It has also been used to break recent peripheral anterior synechiae secondary to an episode of angle closure.

ALPI can be used in cases of chronic angle apposition, to obtain a more open angle, as in cases of iris plateau, nanopthalmos, irido-ciliary cysts, retinopathy of prematurity, and prersistent hyperplastic primary vitreous.[5-9]

ALPI involves placing a series of relatively large, shallow burns on the peripheral iris, as close to the iris root as possible. It causes a thermal shinkage of the collagen fibre structure of the iris, opening a narrow angle.[10]

Unlike laser iridotomy, ALPI does not prevent future attacks, so once the acute attack is past and the cornea has cleared, a laser iridotomy (either argon or yag) is necessary in PACG to prevent future attacks, usually in both eyes.

Periodic gonioscopy should be done to detect further angle closure, indicating a repetition of the ALPI, to prevent trabecular damage, formation of PAS and chronic angle-closure glaucoma.

REFERENCES

1. Mitrev, P.V., Schuman, J.S., Lasers in Glaucoma Management, Focal Points, Vol. XIX No 9, Sept 2001.

2. Preferred Practice Patterns: Primary Angle Closure; American Academy of Ophthalmology, 2000.

3. Ritch R, Liebermann, JM. Laser iridotomy and peripheral iridoplasty. In: Ritch R, Shields MB, Krupin T eds. The Glaucomas, 2nd ed. St. Louis: Mosby, 1996; III: 1549-73.

4. Ritch R: Argon Laser Treatment for Medically Unresponsive Attacks of Angle-Closure Glaucoma; Am J Ophth, 94:197-204, 1982.

5. Lam, DSC; Lai, JSM; Tham,CY: Immediate Argon Laser Peripheral Iridoplasty as Treatment for Acute Attack of Primary Angle-Closure Glaucoma; Ophthalmology, Vol. 105, No 12, Dec. 1998.

6. Ritch R: Argon laser peripheral iridoplasty: an overview. J Glaucoma, 1992;1: 206-13.

7. Saw, SM, Gazzard, G, Friedman, DS: Interventions for Angle-Closure Glaucoma, An Evidence-Based Update; Ophthalmology, Vol. 110, No 10 October 2003.

8. Ritch, R, Chang, BM, Liebmann, JM; Angle Closure in Younger Patients; Ophthalmology, Vol. 110, No 10 October 2003.

9. Wand M: Argon laser gonioplasty for synechial angle closure. Arch Ophthalmol, 1992; 110:363-7.

10. Sassani JW, Ritch R, McCormick S et al: Histopathology of argon laser peripheral iridoplasty. Ophthalmic Surg, 1993; 24:740-5.

Question 47

What are the indications for trabeculectomy in the management of the glaucoma patient?

Jeffrey M. Liebmann

Glaucoma is a pressure-sensitive optic neuropathy characterized by progressive injury to retinal ganglion cells and their axons, changing optic disc topography, and corresponding visual function damage. Pressure-dependent and pressure-independent risk factors contribute to disease onset and progression. Recent evidence from prospective, multi-center, clinical trials assessing the full spectrum of glaucoma diagnoses and disease severity, including early disease (Ocular Hypertension Treatment Study), high-pressure glaucoma (Collaborative Initial Glaucoma Treatment Study), normal-pressure glaucoma (Collaborative Normal Tension Glaucoma Treatment Study), moderate glaucoma (Early Manifest Glaucoma Trial), and advanced glaucoma (Advanced Glaucoma Intervention Study) support the role of IOP reduction as the sole basis of anti-glaucoma therapy for all types of glaucoma and across the diagnostic spectrum. At the present time there is scant, if any, evidence to support any alternative form of therapy.

Reduction of intraocular pressure in glaucoma can be achieved with medications, laser surgery or incisional surgery. The risk and benefits of each form of intervention dictate how each is used. In general, initial antiglaucoma therapy is begun with topical medicines. Medicines, for the most part, offer miminal, reversible risk, and the chance to achieve a moderate pressure reduction. Laser surgery offers the ability to provide modest reduction of IOP without significant side effects, although the result is transient for many patients.. Incisional surgery, usually in the form of trabeculectomy, provides the best means of providing a significant lowering of IOP, although the short-term and long-term risks are greater than medicines or laser surgery.

Assessment of the risk-benefit ratio is one of the most difficult tasks for the surgeon. In glaucoma, consideration must be given to the initial, untreated IOP, the IOP at which the glaucoma damage has progressed, the extent of glaucomatous injury, the ability of the patient to comply with a prescribed antiglaucoma regimen, and the likelihood of significant loss of vision during the patient's lifetime. Increasing life expectancy worldwide suggests that lower target intraocular pressures may be necessary to preserve vision for the lifetime of many patients.

The decision to proceed to trabeculectomy should be made in consultation between the patient and ophthalmologist.. For patients experiencing progressive optic nerve and/or visual field loss, a further target IOP reduction of 30-50% may be required to prevent further loss. Few patients will reach this goal with modification of their medical regimen alone (with or without laser trabeculoplasty) and trabeculectomy is typically indicated. A more difficult decision involves the patient that appears to be clinically stable, but with an IOP that is likely too high for long-term preservation of visual function. A good relationship between the doctor and patient will facilitate a successful surgical outcome.

The early and delayed risks of trabeculectomy impact the decision-making process. The early complications of trabeculectomy (shallow anterior chamber, transient hypotony, etc.) are usually self-limited. The long-term complications of filtering surgery such as cataract, bleb leak, bleb dysesthesia, and bleb-related ocular infection can be quite serious and the patient and the physician need to understand the full impact of trabeculectomy on both the status of the disease and the patient's quality of life.

Surgery should be performed utilizing techniques to minimize risk of complications. This includes careful preoperative evaluation to assess the best surgical technique to minimize anesthesia, intraoperative complications and postoperative hypotony, early detection and timely, appropriate management of complications if they should arise, and management of bleb formation to maximize the chance of successful surgery.

Lastly, the decision to proceed to surgery must be individualized for each patient. The decision to proceed to surgery, either early or late in the disease process, should reflect the practical reality of the advantages and disadvantages of surgery for that particular individual. For some persons without access to expensive medications, surgery might be the best initial treatment modality, while for others, the slow rate of disease progression with medical therapy may eliminate the need for surgical intervention completely.

Question 48

When to use prophylactic antibiotics prior to trabeculectomy?

Daniel Grigera

Most of the available information comes from the field of cataract surgery and we may apply it, not without certain reservations, to glaucoma surgery.

Although antibiotic treatment is more effective than no treatment in sterilizing the external ocular adnexa[1] there is no evidence to support the use of antibiotics prior to trabeculectomy[2,3,4] in all eyes.

Whether to use preoperative antibiotics or not in patients under some risk of infection is subject to controversy.

I personally do it in such cases as nasolacrimal duct obstruction 2%[5] blepharitis[6], conjunctivitis, upper respiratory infection,[7] and specially on patients under immunosuppressive treatment[8]. And, last but not least, when there is an enucleated fellow eye with a prosthesis.

REFERENCES

1. Kirsch LS, Jackson WB, Goldstein DA, Discepola MJ Perioperative ofloxacin vs. to-bramycin: efficacy in external ocular adnexal sterilization and anterior chamber penetration.. Can J Ophthalmol, 1995 Feb;30(1):11-20.

2. Montan PG, Setterquist H, Marcusson E, Rylander M, Ransjo U.Preoperative gentamicin eye drops and chlorhexidine solution in cataract surgery. Experimental and clinical results. Eur J Ophthalmol, 2000 Oct-Dec;10(4):286-92.

3. Colleaux KM, Hamilton WK.Effect of prophylactic antibiotics and incision type on the incidence of endophthalmitis after cataract surgery. Can J Ophthalmol, 2000 Dec; 35(7):373-8.

4. Chitkara DK, Manners T, Chapman F, Stoddart MG, Hill D, Jenkins D.Lack of effect of preoperative norfloxacin on bacterial contamination of anterior chamber aspirates after cataract surgery. Br J Ophthalmol, 1994 Oct;78(10):772-4.

5. Song A, Scott IU, Flynn HW Jr, Budenz DL.Delayed-onset bleb-associated endophthalmitis: clinical features and visual acuity outcomes. Ophthalmology, 2002 May; 109(5):985-91.

6. Mac I, Soltau JB.Glaucoma-filtering bleb infections. Curr Opin Ophthalmol, 2003 Apr; 14(2):91-4.

7. Ashkenazi I, Melamed S, Avni I, Bartov E, Blumenthal M.Risk factors associated with late infection of filtering blebs and endophthalmitis. Ophthalmic Surg, 1991 Oct; 22(10):570-4.

8. Montan PG, Koranyi G, Setterquist HE, Stridh A, Philipson BT, Wiklund K.Endophthalmitis after cataract surgery: risk factors relating to technique and events of the operation and patient history: a retrospective case-control study. Ophthalmology, 1998 Dec; 105(12):2171-7.

Question 49

When and how is 5-fluorouracil (5-FU) used with trabeculectomy?

Robert Feldman

Long-term intraocular pressure (IOP) control, after trabeculectomy may be limited by scarring, generally occurring at the episcleral level. Adjunctive 5FU increases the success rate of trabeculectomy, both in primary and complicated glaucomas by inhibiting fibroblast proliferation and the resulting episcleral fibrosis in the early postoperative period.

5FU is a halogenated pyrimidine analogue, a strong antimetabolite, and an effective antifibrotic agent. This agent converted into a nucleated analog, 5fluoro-2-deoxyuridylate mono phosphates competitively inhibits an enzyme involved in DNA synthesis during the synthesis phase (S phase) of the cell cycle. Abnormal protein products are produced within the cell leading to cell death. All actively dividing cells (those in the S phase of the cell cycle) that come in contact with that agent are affected.

Another antifibrotic agent frequently used is mitomycin C (MMC), which also inhibits DNA synthesis and is applied once during trabeculectomy to the operated site. In concentrations ranging from 0.2-0.5 mg/ml MMC is 100 times more potent in its anti proliferative action than 5FU.

A review by Rothman et al[1] of the survival curves of trabeculectomy revealed that 5FU is effective in decreasing the likely hood of failure within the first 3 years. After 3 years it appears that the failure curve is parallel to trabeculectomy performed without antifibrotics. Khaw et al[2] demonstrated that 5 minutes of intraoperative application of 5FU resulted in a delay of fibroblast proliferation from treated sub conjunctival and scleral tissue for more than one week in a rabbit model, while MMC resulted in prolonged inhibition for at least 30 days.

Spiegel et al[3] postulated that the ability of 5FU to decrease IOP in the early postoperative period may be due not only to its anti metabolite effect, but to a direct toxic effect. Merriman et al[4] in his in vitro study suggested that 1-minute exposure to 5FU had a significant antiproliferative effect on fibroblast of Tenon's capsule, which was similar to 5 minutes of exposure; this has yet to be evaluated clinically.

The use of antifibrotics varies widely among surgeons. Application should be based on the surgeon's perception of likel hood of failure of the surgery and the need for lower intraocular pressures. In some cases no antifibrotic is needed: elderly Caucasian patients with early to moderate disease, and those in which the IOP lowering effect of surgery is needed as a temporizing measure (glaucoma secondary to hyphema). Most others require some antifibrotic regimen either 5FU or MMC.

In the initial studies on 5FU in high-risk eyes frequent postoperative subconjunctival injections were used. The benefit was demonstrated in the 5-year follow up of the Fluorouracil filtration study (Parrish et al[5]). Despite successful IOP control at 1 year, trabeculectomies with 5FU injections fail over time with disappointing success rates of 61% at 1 year, 44% at 10 years and 41% at 14years[6]. Two prospective randomized clinical trails[7,8] have shown that intraoperative MMC application via sponge might be a more beneficial adjunct to trabeculectomy than postoperative 5FU injections in-patient at high risk for failure. In addition, the discomfort of injections, the inconvenience to both patient and physician and the frequent corneal side effect led to the use of intraoperative 5FU.

5FU used intraoperatively is now the antifibrotic of choice in primary trabeculectomy in low risk eyes without any of the following characteristics: secondary glaucomas (excluding pigmentary and pseudoexfoliation) childhood glaucomas, non-compliant patients, normal tension glaucoma and previous surgery involving the conjunctiva or the need for low target pressures (normal tension glaucoma or severely advanced disease). Some authors also believe that black race is a risk factor requiring MMC.

Intraoperative 5FU eases suture lysis; the resulting bleb is thinner with less conjunctival injection, making the scleral flap sutures more easily visible. By delaying wound healing suture lysis can be effective for up to three weeks postoperatively.

Singh et al[9] reported that with intra operative 5FU, fewer postoperative injections and resultant fewer side effects could be administered without a reduction in success compared to trabeculectomy with postoperative 5FU injections only.

Anand[10] and Watts et al[11] demonstrated that single, low dose intraoperative administration of 5FU is adequate to obtain IOP's in the low teens in low risk eyes. However intra operative 5FU alone may not be enough in moderate or high-risk eyes.

Feldman et al[12] used high dose 5FU (50mg/ml) for 5 minutes in a single application during filtration surgery and found it safe in low-moderate risk eyes, but not effective in high-risk eyes. The success rate in six months follow up in low risk eyes was 92%, in moderate risk eyes 88% and in high-risk eyes 57%. Mora[13] and Sidoti et al[14] also reported that high dose intra operative 5FU is effective and safe adjunct in trabeculectomy, but high-risk eyes may require supplemental postoperative 5FU injections.

At the present time, 5FU is given in low risk trabeculectomy as an intraoperative dose of 50 mg/ml for 5 minutes based on data (unpublished results) using radio labeled 5FU in cadaver eyes to determine time to maximum tissue concentrations.

The importance of intra operative 5FU has become clear over years of patient care but sometimes it is not enough and post-operative 5FU injections should be given based on the appearance of the bleb, even in cases where MMC was used intraoperatively.

For injected blebs and those that appear thickened within the first two weeks post- operatively, subconjunctival injections may be useful in doses of 5 to 7.5 mg adjacent to the bleb[15].

5FU has also been used as an adjunct to needle revision of the bleb. Shin[16] and Hawkins et al[17] reported a success rate of the initial 5FU needling revision, was 45% at 1 year, 33% at 2 years, and 28% at 4 years. Needling failure correlated with pre needling IOP > 30 mmHg, lack of MMC during the previous filtration surgery, and IOP > 10 mmHg immediately after needling revision, also fornix-based trabeculectomies were more likely to fail needle revision than limbus-based trabeculectomies.

The role of 5FU compared to MMC has been extensively evaluated and has led to the intraoperative use of 5FU being limited to low risk eyes as described above. Smith et al[18] demonstrated that 50 mg/ml 5FU for 5 minutes and MMC 0.2 mg/ml for 3-5 minutes both can provide good intermediate term IOP control and may be used in eyes requiring final target IOP's in low teens or single digits. Singh[19] and Wudunn et al[20] compared 5FU 50mg/ml for 5 minutes to MMC 0.4 mg/ml for 2 minutes and found that both are safe and effective in primary trabeculectomy in eyes not at high risk for failure, in the short and medium term. Vijaya et al[21] stated that low dose intra operative MMC (0.2, 0.4mg/ml) and 5FU (50mg/ml) for one minute can control IOP in primary trabeculectomy but 5FU resulted in fewer-ischemic blebs which may be an indicator of late complications (bleb leaks, hypotony and infections). Therefore, MMC should be reserved for higher-risk eyes.

Many surgeon dependent variables (application method, timing, rinsing the anti metabolites, limbus versus fornix based conjunctival flap, conjunctiva closure technique the sponge size, type and brand, the concentration and the volume of the anti fibrotic agents) may result in differing success rates with intraoperative anti metabolites. Previous work has evaluated the absorption and release of MMC by surgical spears[22], Merocel sponge spears (Medtronic Solan Ophthalmic Product Inc., Jacksonville, FL, U.S.A) were shown to absorb significantly more solution than the other brands including Weck-cell (Medtronic Solan Ophthalmic Product Inc., Jacksonville, FL, U.S.A) but not Altomed (Altomed Ltd., Boldon, England, U.K), however saturated Weck-cell spears released more solution when placed on filter paper than did the others.

Wilkins et al[23] investigated the effect of sponge type and brand on tissue levels of 5FU in an experimental model (pig eyes) and found that Altomed (Altomed Ldt., U.K) sponges deliver significantly more radiolabelled 5FU than Weck-Cell (Medtronic Solan Inc., U.S.A) or Merocel (Medtronic Solan Inc., U.S.A) sponges and diluting the 25mg/ml 5FU solution by factor of 4 significantly reduces the conjunctival levels by factor of 4, he also reports that replacing a sponge every minute for 5 minutes did not improve conjunctival and scleral levels compared with applying a single sponge for 5 minutes. Also, changing the size of the sponge does not increase the tissue levels of 5FU either. However, Brook et al[24] suggested that most trabeculectomy techniques could be effective with intraoperative 5FU.

Postoperative complications related to the 5FU administration as it is done today are unusual:

- Persistent choroidal effusions

- Corneal epithelial defects
- Sub conjunctival hemorrhages (injection site)
- Hyphema
- Persistent wound leaks and wound dehiscences
- Persistent hypotony (IOP<5mmHg more than 3 months after surgery)
- Increased rate of bleb related infections

Differences in rates of complications between 5FU and MMC reported have been controversial but most believe that MMC results in more leaky ischemic blebs, hypotony and infection while 5FU results in more corneal epithelial defects.

In summary intraoperative 5FU should be considered in low risk eyes not needing very low target IOPs and as postoperative adjunctive therapy in eyes with blebs that appear to be at risk for failure. MMC should be reserved for higher risk eyes in which the associated greater complication rate is acceptable.

REFERENCES

1. Rothman R.F., Liebmann J.M., Ritch R. Low-dose 5-fluorouracil trabeculectomy as initial surgery in uncomplicated glaucoma: long-term follow up. Ophthalmology, 2000; 107:1184-1190.

2. Khaw P.T., Doyle J.W, Sherwood M.B., Grierson I., Schultz G., McGorray S. Prolong localized tissue effect from 5-minute exposure to fluorouracil and mitomycin C. Arch Ophthalmol, 1993;111:263-267.

3. Spiegel D., Sachs H., Yanes G. Single dose intraoperative administration of 5-fluorouracil in trabeculectomy. Long-term result of a pilot study. Ophthalmology, 1996:93:561-566.

4. Merriman M, Mora J, Beaumont B, Merrilees M. Effects of varying 5FY exposure duration on tenon's capsule fibroblasts. Clin Experiment Ophthalmol, 2001;29:248-52.

5. Five-year follow-up of the fluorouracil filtering surgery study. The fluorouracil study group. Am j. Ophthalmol, 1996;121:349-66.

6. Susuki R, Dickens CJ, Iwach A, Hoskins H et al. Long-term follow-up of initially successful trabeculectomy with 5FU injections. Ophthalmol, 2002;109:1921-4.

7. Kitazawa Y, Kawase K, Matsushita H, Minobi M. Trabeculectomy with MMC. A comparative study with fluorouracil. Arch Ophthalmol, 1991;109:1693-8.

8. Skuta GL, Beeson CC, Hagginbotham EJ et al. Intraoperative mitomycin versus postoperative %FU in high-risk glaucoma filtering surgery. Ophthalmol, 1992;99:438-444.

9. Singh R, Goldberg I, Mohsin M. The efficacy and safety of intraoperative and/or postoperative 5FU in trabeculectomy and phacotrabeculectomy. Clin Experiment Ophthalmol, 2001;29:296-302.

10. Anand N., Sahni K., Menage MJ. Modification of trabeculectomy with single-dose intraoperative 5-fluorouracil application. Acta Ophthalmol Scand, 1998;76:83-89.

11. Watts P., Karia N., McAllister J. Is the single use of intraoperative 5FU in filtering surgery for high-risk cases enough? Eye, 1998;12:374-8.

12. Feldman RM, Dietze PJ, Gross RL, Oram O. Intra operative 5-fluorouracil administration in trabeculectomy. J Glaucoma, 1994;3:302-307.

13. Mora JS, Nguyen N, Iwach AG, Gaffiney MM, Hetherington J Jr., Hoskins HD, Wong PC, Tran H, Dickens CJ. Trabeculectomy with intra operative sponge 5-fluorouracil. Ophthalmol, 1996;103:963-970.

14. Sidoti PA, Choi JC, Morinelli EN, Lee PP, Baerveldt G, Minckler DS, Heuer DK. Trabeculectomy with intra operative 5-fluorouracil. Ophthalmic Surg Lasers, 1998; 29:552-561.

15. Weinreb. Adjusting the dose of 5FU after filtration surgery to minimize side effects. Ophthalmol, 1987;94:564-70.

16. Shin D, Kim Y, Ginde S, Kim P et al. risk factors for failure of 5FU needling revision for failed conjunctival filtration blebs. AM J.Ophthalmol, 2001;132:875-80.

17. Hawkins A, Flanagan J, Brown S. Predictors for success of needle revision of failing filtration blebs. Ophthalmol, 2002;109:781-5.

18. Smith MF, Doyle JW, Nguyen QH, Sherwood MB. Results of intra operative 5-fluorouracil or lower dose mitomycin-C administration on initial trabeculectomy surgery. J Glaucoma, 1997;6:104-110.

19. Singh K, Mehta K, Shaikh N, Tsai J, Moster M et al. Trabeculectomy with intraoperative mitomycin versus 5FU. Ophthalmol, 2000;107:2305-2309.

20. WuDunn D, Cantor LB, Palanca-Capistrano AM, Hoop J, Alvi NP, Finley C, Lakhani V, Burnstein A, Knotts SL. A prospective randomized trial comparing intra operative 5-fluorouracil vs. mitomycin-C in primary trabeculectomy. Am J Ophthalmol, 2002; 134:521-528.

21. Vijaya L, Mukhesh B, Shantha B et al. comparison of low-dose intra operative MMC vs. 5FU in primary glaucoma surgery: a pilot study. Ophthalmic Surg Lasers, 2000; 31:24-30.

22. Flynn W, Carlson D, Biffano S. Mitomycin trabeculectomy: the microsurgical difference. J.Glaucoma, 1995;4:86-90.

23. Wilkins MR, Occlestone NL, Kotecha A, Waters L, Khaw PT. Sponge delivery variables and tissue levels of 5-fluorouracil. Br J Ophthalmol, 2000;84:92-97.

24. Brook AM, Gillies WE. Design and results of trabeculectomy operation for use with 5-fluorouracil. Ophthalmic Surg, 1992;23:242-245.

Question 50

When and how is mitomycin C used with trabeculectomy?

P. T. Khaw

Introduction

Agents which modulate healing such as the anti-metabolites 5-fluorouracil (5FU) and mitomycin-c (MMC) have revolutionised glaucoma surgery, in patients with a high risk of surgical failure. There is increasing evidence from long term prospective trials, that intraocular pressures in the 10 –15 mmHg range best preserve long term vision in glaucoma.[1;2] However, vision threatening complications occur with the use of these agents.[3;4]

Changes in clinical techniques of antimetabolite application can increase the safety and considerably reduce complications while maintaining effectiveness. In this chapter I will describe how our surgical technique has been changed to make the use of antimetabolites as safe as possible – the Safe Surgery System. This technique has evolved at Moorfields based on both clinical observation and experimental studies to reduce complications and enhance success. Some changes in surgical technique are necessary to take full advantage of these improvements. The techniques and materials described are straightforward and have been designed to be easily available to ophthalmologists.

Which antifibrotic agent

There are many antifibrosis agents available for use and these range from steroids used in virtually every patient, through to antimetabolites and newer experimental agents. The indications for different agents are too extensive for this chapter and are covered elsewhere[5]. Details of this and all

227

the techniques described is this chapter Can be downloaded from:
http://www.ucl.ac.uk/ioo/research/khaw.htm

Application technique

The variations in the technique used to deliver intraoperative antimetabolites may account for some of the variations in efficacy and complications seen in the literature. It is very important for individual users to maintain a consistent technique and to build up experience with one technique.

Changes in area of treatment, conjunctival and scleral flap construction, and adjustable sutures have led to a dramatic difference in terms of reducing short and long term complications. (Figure 1 and 2) This has led to a reduction in cystic areas within the bleb from 90% to 29%. The blebitis and endophthalmitis rate over 3-5 years was 20% for older limbus based techniques with a smaller treatment area versus 0% over the same period for the current technique.[6] Falls in complication rate have also been seen in the USA in lower risk populations from approximately 6% to 0.5% to date (Paul Palmberg personal communication) If these figures were extrapolated

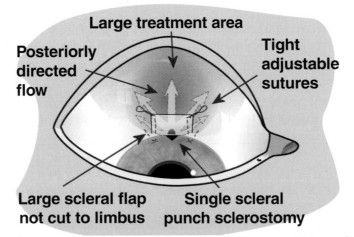

Figure 1. Technique changes associated with antimetabolites use which result in more diffuse non-cystic blebs which are much less likely to develop long term complications and more controlled surgery "Safe Surgery System".

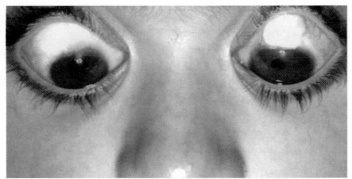

Figure 2. Difference in bleb appearance in left eye (Limbus based conjunctival flap, small scleral flap and smaller area of MMC 0.4 mg/ml treatment) versus right eye (Fornix based flap, larger scleral flap and larger area of MMC 0.5 mg/ml treatment).

to an approximate figure of 50,000 trabeculectomies with antimetabolite per year in the United States it is possible that bleb related complications could be avoided in many thousands of patients.

1) *Intraoperative application of antimetabolite*

Type of incision/dissection

I have changed to a fornix-based incision for either intraoperative 5FU or MMC. The cut length is approximately 8mm. I do not make a relieving incision to avoid any restricting incision. I dissect backwards with Westcott scissors to make a pocket of approximately 10-15mm posteriorly and wide for the antimetabolite sponges. When I dissect over the superior rectus tendon. I lift the conjunctiva to cut attachments avoiding the tendon itself (Figure 3).

Explanation: I always previously used a limbus-based incision with antimetabolite as I was worried about postoperative leaks. However, my clinical observation of cystic blebs led me to the hypothesis that they had two things in common. The first was restricted posterior flow "the ring of steel". The second was anterior aqueous flow. Even cystic blebs from preantimetabolite days have these.

The restricted flow from the posterior incision resulting in more focal cystic blebs led me to change. The effects of treatment are very focal [7;8] and the cells at the edge of the treatment area although growth arrested [9;10] and can make scar tissue and encapsulate the area resulting in thinning and a cystic bleb. A fornix-based incision allows a larger area of antimetabolite treatment, without a posteriorly placed restricting scar.

Similar blebs can be achieved with a limbus-based flap but the incision has to be very posteriorly placed and this result is not as consistent. This does make the subsequent scleral flap and sutures more difficult.

Scleral flap

I now cut the scleral flap before I apply antimetabolite. I try to cut the largest flap possible and leave the side cuts at the limbus incomplete (1-2 mm from limbus). This forces the aqueous backwards over a wider area to get a diffuse bleb.

Explanation. An aqueous jet at the limbus predisposes to an anterior focal cystic bleb, whereas posteriorly directed diffuse flow of aqueous from incompletely cut sides of a large scleral flap results in a more diffuse non-cystic bleb. There is also evidence that treatment under the flap increases the success rate.[11] Finally, if dissection occurs before the antimetabolite treatment, if there is any defect in the flap the use of intraoperative agents particularly mitomycin can be avoided and postoperative injections used instead.

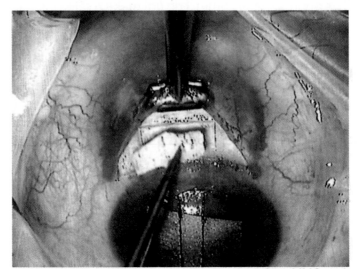

Figure 3. T clamp used to lift conjunctiva and keep edge away from MMC soaked sponges.

Conjunctival clamp

I use a special conjunctival T clamp I designed (Duckworth and Kent 2-686 Duckworthand Kent.com) to hold back the conjunctiva and to prevent antimetabolite touch. This clamp maintains a pocket for antimetabolite treatment. (Figure 3)

Explanation: Our experiments have shown that the antimetabolite affects mainly the area it touches, }[8] therefore protecting the edge prevents wound leaks and dehiscence.

Type of sponge

I use circular medical grade polyvinyl alcohol sponges used for Lasik and corneal shileds rather than other sponges. I cut the sponges in half. Fold nthem like a foldable lens and they fit through the entrance to the pocket without touching the sides (approximately 5 mm X 3 and insert about 6 of these). I attempt to treat as large an area as I can. I also treat under the scleral flap.

I have used polyvinyl alcohol sponges for many years as they maintain their integrity and do not fragment. In contrast, other sponges (e.g. Weck Cell) fragment relatively easily, with an increased chance of leaving small pieces of sponge behind in the wound. The large area of treatment results in more diffuse non-cystic blebs clinically. I treat under the flap as there is evidence that it improves the success rate. In addition when I have re-explored failed surgery I have found adhesions between the scleral flap and bed in addition to episcleral fibrosis.

Increasing the surface area of treatment results in a much more diffuse non-cystic area clinically. A large area prevents the development of a ring of scar tissue (the "ring of Steel") which restricts flow and promotes the development of a raised cystic avascular bleb.

Antimetabolite treatment duration and washout.

I treat for three minutes. If I need to vary the effect of MMC I vary the concentration. I use only two concentrations (0.2 and 0.5 mg/ml) For intraoperative 5FU I always use 50mg/ml. I washout with 20 ml of balanced salt solution.

Explanation: Pharmacokinetic experiments we have done show a rapid uptake over three minutes after which there is a plateau when relatively little drug is added for extra minutes. In the period from 1 to 3 minutes there is considerable variation in the dose delivered.[12]

Scleral flap sutures - New adjustable, releaseable and fixed

The sclerostomy is created and secured with a mixture of fixed and releaseable sutures. I have also developed a new type of adjustable suture which I have now evolved for about 2 years. These allow the tension to be adjusted post operatively through the conjunctiva. Specially designed forceps with very smooth edges are used for this adjustment of pressure. (Duckworth and Kent 2-502) (Figure 4).

Explanation: If strong antimetabolites such as MMC are used complete suture removal can lead to a sudden drop in intraocular pressure even many months after surgery. An adjustable suture system allows a gradual titration of the intraocular pressure – more gradual than that seen with suture removal or massage.[13]

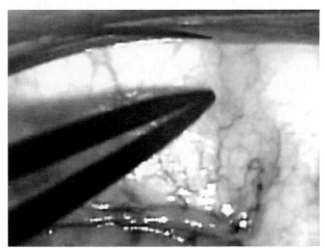

Figure 4. Special adjustable suture forceps being used to adjust pressure down slowly through onjunctiva.

Conjunctival closure

The main reason fornix based flaps are not popular despite the increased speed, much better exposure and absence of a scar in the line of aqueous flow leading to more cystic blebs is the inconvenience of aqueous leakage at the limbus in the post operative period. To get round this problem and take advantage of a fornix based bleb we have used several strategies

- No side cut in the conjunctiva – this minimises manipulation and side leakage

- Ensure Tenons is engaged in every stitch rather than just conjunctiva

- Minimise any contact with antimetabolites e.g. with clamp

- Side purse string sutures and deep attachment sutures buried in corneal grooves. 10/0 nylon is used throughout.

2) *Postoperative application of antimetabolites*

I do not give routine subconjunctival injections of MMC because of the risks Injections of 5FU can be used post operatively. Again the technique of injection may be very important. Our laboratory experiments show that the degree of effect of antimetabolites on fibroblasts depends on either concentration or duration of exposure hence the logic for using a very high concentration of 5FU intraoperatively in the surgical area. [8;14]

It is logical to deliver the injection of 5FU as close as possible to the bleb, but without entering the bleb itself. Delivered this way, injections may be needed much less frequently than previously. However, it is vital that 5FU does not enter the eye as apart from its antimetabolite action, commercial 5FU has a pH of approximately 9, and great care should be taken particularly in a soft eye. It may be useful to washout the fornix shortly after injection. We have developed a new technique of 5-FU preceded by subconjunctival Haelon GV[TM]. This prevents leakage of 5FU back into the tear film and enhances the effect of the 5-FU (Figure 5).

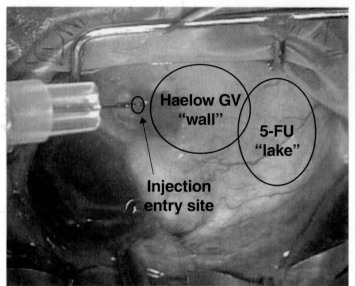

Figure 5. Technique of subconjunctival injection of 5-FU with Haelon GV to prevent 5FU tear film reflux and increase effect of 5FU.

Summary

Simple changes in the method of intraoperative antimetabolite application coupled with changes in surgical technique can very greatly increase the long-term safety of filtration surgery. (Figure 6).

Acknowledgements

Our research has been supported in part by the Medical Research Council (G9330070), the Guide Dogs for the Blind, the Wellcome Trust, the RNIB, Eranda Trust, Hayman Trust, Moorfields Trustees, the Healing Fund, Ronald Liora Moskovitz and the Michael and Ilse Katz Foundation, who have supported our glaucoma and ocular repair and regneration research programme. Without them newer safer techniques for surgery would not have been developed. Mr Alan Lacey produced the diagrams.

The author has no financial interest in any of the products listed in this review including the instruments which he has designed.

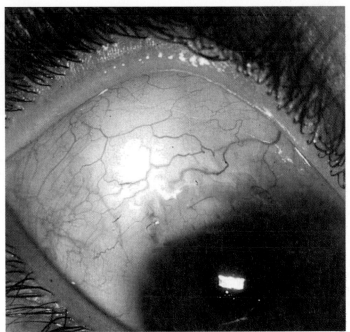

Figure 6. Diffuse non-cystic bleb with a pressure of 11 mmHg following surgery with intraoperative MMC 0.5 mg/ml. This result may be possible for the majority of patients having filtration surgery with improvements of current techniques, and can lead to a dramatic reduction in complications.

REFERENCES

1. The Advanced Glaucoma Intervention Study (AGIS): 7. The relationship between control of intraocular pressure and visual field deterioration.The AGIS Investigators. Am J Ophthalmol, 2000; 2000 Oct;130:429-40.

2. The effectiveness of intraocular pressure reduction in the treatment of normal-tension glaucoma. Collaborative Normal-Tension Glaucoma Study Group. Am J Ophthalmol, 1998; 1998 Oct;126:498-505.

3. Higginbotham EJ, Stevens RK, Musch DC, Karp KO, Lichter PR, Bergstrom TJ *et al*. Bleb-related endophthalmitis after trabeculectomy with mitomycin C. 8 1996; 1996 Apr;103:650-6.

4. Greenfield DS, Suner IJ, Miller MP, Kangas TA, Palmberg PF, Flynn HW. Endophthalmitis after filtering surgery with mitomycin. Arch Ophthalmol, 1996; 1996 Aug; 114:943-9.

5. Khaw PT, Chang LPY. Antifibrotic agents in glaucoma surgery. In Duker D, Yanoff.M., eds. Ophthalmology - a practical textbook., London: Churchill Livingston, 2003.

6. Wells, A. P., Cordeiro, M. F., Bunce, C., and Khaw, P. T. Cystic bleb formation and related complications in limbus versus fornix based flaps in paediatric and young adult trabeculectomy with mitomycin-C. Ophthalmology, 110, 2192-2197. 2003.

7. Khaw PT, Doyle JW, Sherwood MB, Grierson I, Schultz G, McGorray S. Prolonged localized tissue effects from 5-minute exposures to fluorouracil and mitomycin C. Arch Ophthalmol, 1993; 1993 Feb;111:263-7.

8. Khaw PT, Sherwood MB, MacKay SLD, Rossi MJ, Schultz G. 5-Minute Treatments with Fluorouracil, Floxuridine and Mitomycin Have Long-Term Effects on Human Tenon's Capsule Fibroblasts. Arch Ophthalmol, 1992;110:1150-4.

9. Occleston NL, Daniels JT, Tarnuzzer RW, Sethi KK, Alexander RA, Bhattacharya SS *et al.* Single exposures to antiproliferatives: long-term effects on ocular fibroblast wound-healing behavior. Invest Ophthalmol Vis Sci, 1997; 38:1998-2007.

10. Daniels JT, Occleston NL, Crowston JG, Khaw PT. Effects of antimetabolite induced cellular growth arrest on fibroblast-fibroblast interactions. Exp Eye Res, 1999; 69:117-27.

11. El Sayyad F, Belmekki M, Helal M, Khalil M, El Hamzawey H, Hisham M. Simultaneous subconjunctival and subscleral mitomycin-C application in trabeculectomy, 8 2000; 2000 Feb;107:298-301.

12. Wilkins MR, Occleston NL, Kotecha A, Waters L, Khaw PT. Sponge delivery variables and tissue levels of 5-fluorouracil. Br J Ophthalmol, 2000; 2000 Jan;84:92-7.

13. Wells, A. P., Bunce, C., and Khaw, P. T. Flap and suture manipulation after trabeculectomy with adjustable sutures : Titration of flow intraocular pressure in guarded filtration surgery. J Glaucoma, 2003. In Press.

14. Khaw PT, Ward S, Porter A, Grierson I, Hitchings RA, Rice NSC. The long-term effects of 5-fluorouracil and sodium butyrate on human Tenon's fibroblasts. Invest Ophthalmol Vis Sci, 1992;33:2043-52.

Question 51

When should we use releasable sutures in trabeculectomies?

Heryberto S. Alvim

L. Jay Katz

Introduction

Trabeculectomy has become the most common filtration procedure for glaucoma primarily because it produces fewer postoperative complications than any of the full thickness drainage surgeries [1]. During trabeculectomies the surgeon attempts to achieve two different goals: suture the scleral flap tight enough to prevent overfiltration in the postoperative period, but loose enough to permit proper aqueous humor outflow.

In order to titrate filtration postoperatively, many surgeons advocate tight closure of the scleral flap, with postoperative sutures lysis with an argon or diode laser as elevated IOP develops [2]. This is an often utilized effective approach, but it requires a special lens, access to a laser, and in certain instances is not possible to perform (Figures 1 and 2). Intra- or subconjunctival hemorrhage or a thickened Tenon's layer may obscure the view of the sutures. The patient often has a sensitive eye in the first 1-2 weeks after surgery making this procedure potentially uncomfortable.

Description of the releasable suture techniques

An alternative to laser lysis are the releasable sutures. This technique has been developed and popularized by different surgeons such as Wilson, Cohen *et al*, Shin, Johnstone *et al*, and Hsu and Maberley *et al* [3-7,9]. The procedures are performed identical to a standard trabeculectomy except for

237

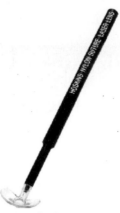

Figure 1. Hoskins lenses for laser suture lysis.

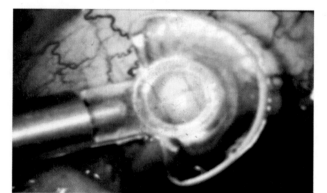

Figure 2. Laser suture lysis or cut/remove releasable sutures with the Hoskins lens.

the closure of the scleral flap. In all these versions a scleral flap suture is externalized that can be easily released and removed at the slip lamp, without the need for a laser, in the postoperative period. Most of these methods involve leaving a long suture end on the cornea, forming a suture track from the outside to the subconjunctival space. These sutures may be released by transconjunctival lysis [10], by cutting the externalized suture [11], or pulled out by holding the end of a buried hemibow tie [5] .(Figures 3 to 6)

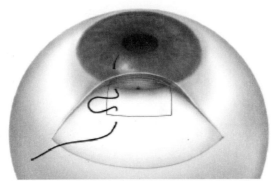

Figure 3. (Cohen and Osher's Technique) First the suture goes through intact sclera to the apex of the scleral flap. Subsequently the needle passes deeply at the base of the flap through the limbus coming out in the clear cornea.

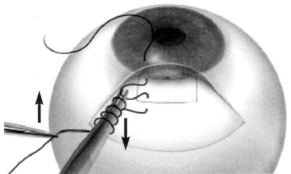

Figure 4. (Cohen and Osher's Technique) At this point a four throw knot is done over the curved forceps forming a loop suture at the apex of the scleral flap.

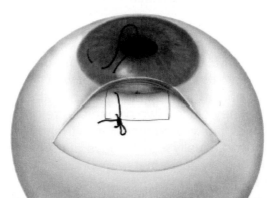

Figure 5. (Cohen and Osher's Technique) A second pass through the stroma is then performed.

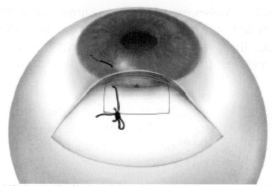

Figure 6. (Cohen and Osher's Technique) A flat loop is left over the epithelium and the end of the suture is cut close to the corneal surface. In this way there is no exposed knot or suture end that would be irritating. Later removal of the suture is accomplished simply by grabbing the elbow of the corneal suture which is the most superficial section and merely pulling to loosen and remove the suture.

Discussion

The great advantage of the releasable sutures is to optimize the IOP in the early postoperative time. It does not seem to affect the final IOP control, but the studies show that the patients do better short-term, especially regarding hypotony related complications. The risk of developing a flat anterior chamber, choroidal effusion, suprachoroidal hemorrhage, aqueous misdirection, and hypotony maculopathy has been markedly lessened by avoiding hypotony with a tighter scleral flap closure with releasable sutures. With a titrated IOP reduction by releasing sutures in the postoperative period filtering surgery success in IOP reduction can be attained without the associated risks with postoperative hypotony.

Kolker *et al* reviewed the charts of 258 patients who had filtering operations form 1988 to 1990, and divided into two groups: one group in which 124 patients had permanent sutures, and the other with 146 cases in which the releasable suture technique was applied. None of these patients received any antimetabolites. They placed two or one suture depending on whether the shape of the scleral flap was rectangular or triangular, respectively. The first suture was removed usually 1 to 10 days after surgery and the second one to seven days later; they noted that removing suture after 14 days had no effect. The results in the group with releasable sutures were encouraging. Only 15% in the study group had shallow anterior chamber compared to 32.8% of the controls (p=.0003). Accordingly, surgical intervention to drain suprachoroidal fluid was also more often required in the control group. The IOP was higher in the study group for the first few days following the trabeculectomy, but then it became similar form day 7 to 1 year, with a similar rate of successes (as defined by IOP reduction) between the two groups.

A modified releasable "U" shaped suture was developed by Maberley et al[9]. In his technique a simple two-arm suture is placed leaving no exposed suture ends. He presented his results in 28 cases. He achieved good IOP control in all cases without any significant complications.

The releasable sutures may be also used when performing combined cataract and glaucoma procedures. Hsu and colleagues [7] compared the outcomes of trabeculectomies and triple procedures (trabeculectomy, extracapsular cataract extraction and posterior chamber lens implantation) with both groups using releasable sutures. In the same study he presents his own modification of releasable sutures using the hemibow tie. The knot is externalized, outside the conjunctiva. In their study the most of the sutures were removed within 4 weeks after surgery. After a mean follow up of 11 months the overall success rate was 78.6%, and there was no significant difference from both surgical groups. As demonstrated in other studies the immediate pressure-lowering effect was greater in the eyes in which the sutures were removed relatively early. Other studies also could demonstrate an IOP decrease with suture release following trabeculectomy alone or combined with a cataract extraction[8].

When to release the suture

Rudimentary guidelines for the timing for release of the suture were based on retrospective studies and also from experience with laser suture lysis .In 1998 Ranita et al [13] published the first prospective, randomized study about releasable sutures. She followed 30 patients for 12 months, divided into two groups: 15 trabeculectomies with conventional interrupted sutures and 15 cases with a releasable suture technique. Antimetabolites were not utilized in either group. In all cases 3 sutures on the scleral flap were applied. A single suture was released every time the IOP rose above 21 mmHg or whenever bleb massage was ineffective. In the short-term, the IOP behaved the same way as in Kolker's study. However, in longer-term follow-up they noticed that the mean IOP at 6 and 12 months in the non-releasable suture group was significant higher. An analysis of the releasable suture group showed that the maximum change in the IOP occurred when sutures were released between days 1 to 5 (34.8% drop), while minimal or no change happened when released between days 11 to 15 (11.5% drop). A moderate change was reported when the sutures were released between days 6 to 10 (33.8%).

Antifibrotics like mitomycin and 5-FU modulate wound healing which has proven invaluable in filtrating procedures especially difficult cases. The delay in the healing process provided by antifibrotics may extend the period for effective releasable suture removal. Extension of the "window of opportunity" has been demonstrated for argon laser suture lysis after trabeculectomy with mitomycin C in which effective laser suture lysis was obtained even when it was performed until 7 to 21 weeks postoperatively [14]. In 1997 Thomas et al[8] did a retrospective review of 154 trabeculectomies to assess the effect of suture release on IOP in various postoperative periods. Fourteen eyes had daily 5-FU injections for 5 to 7 days; another 54 eyes received 0.4mg/ml MMC for three minutes. They could not demonstrate a significant difference in the pressure lowering effect between the eyes with or without adjunctive antimetabolites use. However they show that on suture releases within 21 days, eyes receiving mitomycin C seemed to have a greater mean decrease in IOP (7.6 mmHg) compared to eyes receiving 5-FU (5.3 mmHg), however the difference was not statistically significant. The release after 21 days promoted a fall on IOP of only 2.3 mmHg, what clinically might not be significant.

Tezel et al [15] did a similar study with 324 patients, in whom all cases got antifibrotic therapy (MMC in 534 eyes, and 5-FU in 29 eyes). Postoperative suture removal occurred beyond 3 weeks for at least 1 of the 2 releasable sutures in 147 eyes. The immediate IOP reduction was 6.3 ± 2.8 mmHg, if all sutures removed after 3 weeks are taken together. This study demonstrated a definitive clinical effect in IOP reduction following late releasable suture removal in trabeculectomies and combined procedures supplemented with antifibrotics. However the magnitude of the IOP reduction was inversely correlated with the postoperative interval when the releasable suture was removed. According to Unlu et al [16], after a prospective analysis of 18 patients, concluded that the suture removal at the 4th week had no noticeable effect on the IOP even when MMC is used (change in IOP was 2.21 mmHg), but there was no information about the 3rd to 4th weeks. The difference in the various studies as to whether "late" suture removal can effectively lower the IOP may be variable due to differences in technique such as the scleral flap construction and the number of scleral flap sutures. Regardless of the conflicting results we should assume that the use of antifibrotics allows us to extend the removal time of releasable suture longer then those two weeks established from earlier studies without antimetabolites.

Complications

The releasable suture technique is usually a relatively safe procedure. However it is not free of complications. The externalized suture may serve as a nidus for infection and provide a potential route for organisms to reach the anterior chamber. Burchfield [17] and Rosenberg [18] reported the first cases of postoperative endophthalmitis following trabeculectomy with releasable sutures. A corneal abscess developed around the releasable suture site with intraocular extension. In both cases the end of the suture was not buried and the patients were no longer on topical antibiotics. Based on this information, the surgeon should bury the releasable suture end within the cornea and continue the topical administration of antibiotics for as long as the exposed suture is present. A second cornea pass also reduces the amount of exposed suture and reduces the "windshield wiper effect" another complication related to the technique [8,12,19]. The windshield wiper effect is a corneal epithelial defect that occurs due to the rubbing of the suture on the cornea with the movement of the lids. Its not clear if the use of antifibrotics might increase this finding. An exposed knot may induce a foreign body irritation. The removal of the suture may lead to some other complications such as: aqueous humor leak along the suture tract [12,16], shallowing or even flattening [12,16] of the anterior chamber, suture breakage or failure to release the suture [8,12,15,16,19], subconjunctival hemorrhage [8,12,19]. Most of these complications are conservatively approached with observation since they typically will resolve spontaneously.

Conclusion

Finally, after consideration of the studies cited and clinical experience, we conclude that control of IOP in the early postoperative period with releasable sutures are preferred to reliance on laser lysis of permanent scleral flap sutures. Releasable flap sutures provide a relatively safe adjunct to filtrating procedures. Minimal equipment is required for removal. Only fine tying forceps are needed and removal of the suture can be accomplished at the slit lamp with topical anesthesia. It may be effective with trabeculectomies or combined cataract and glaucoma procedures. When antifibrotic therapy with mitomycin C or 5-fluoruracil is employed the window of opportunity for releasing the suture may be extended beyond 2 weeks. The final success rate in IOP control may not be different than using regular scleral flap sutures, however lessening the complication rate related to the postoperative hypotony is reassuring. With the titration of IOP postoperatively with releasable sutures the surgeon provides a safer more controlled postoperative course for the patient.

REFERENCES

1. Spaeth GL, Joseph NH, Fernandes E: Trabeculectomy: a reevaluation after three years and a comparison with Scheie's procedure. Trans Am Acad Ophthalmol Otolaryngol 1975; 79:349-61.

2. Savage JA, Condon GP, Lyte RA, Simmons RJ. Laser suture lysis after trabeculectomy. Ophthalmology 1988;95:1631.

3. Cohen JS, Osher RH. Releasable scleral flap suture. Ophthalmol Clin North Am 1988, 1:187-97.

4. Wilson RP. Technical advances in filtration surgery. In: McAllister JA, Wilson RP, eds. Glaucoma. Stoneham, mass: Butterworths; 1986:243-50.

5. Shin DH. Removable-suture closure of the lamellar scleral flap in trabeculectomy. Ann Ophthalmol 1987; 19:51-3.

6. Johnstone MA, Wellington DP, Ziel CJ. A releasable scleral flap tamponade suture for guarded filtration surgery. Arch Ophthalmol 1993;111:398-403.

7. Hsu CT, Yarng SS. A modified removable suture in trabeculectomy. Ophthalmic Surg 1993;24:579-85.

8. Thomas R, Jacob, P, Braganza A, et al. Releasable suture technique for trabeculectomy. Indian J Ophthalmol 1997;45:37-41.

9. Maberley D, Apel A, Rootman DS. Releasable "U" suture for trabeculectomy surgery. Ophthalmic Surgery 1994;25(4):251-255.

10. Hoskins HD JR, Migliazzo C. Management of failing filtering blebs with the argon laser. Ophthalmic Surg 1984; 15:731-33.

11. Wilson RP. Releasable sutures in filtration surgery. In Sherwood MB, Spaeth GL, ed. Complications of Glaucoma Therapy. Thorofare, NJ: SLACK Inc; 1990: 199-209.

12. Kolker AE, Kass MA, Rait JL. Trabeculectomy with releasable sutures. Arch Ophthalmol 1994;112:62-6.

13. Ranita UK, Tuli D. Trabeculectomy with releasable sutures. Arch Ophthalmol 1998;116:1288-1293.

14. Pappa KS, Derick RJ, Weber PA, Kapetansky FM, et al. Late argon laser suture lysis after mitomycin C trabeculectomy. Ophthalmology 1993;100:1268-71.

15. Tezel G, Kolker AE, Kass M, Wax MB. Late removal of released sutures after trabeculectomy or combined trabeculectomy with cataract extraction supplemented with antifibrotics. J Glaucoma 1998;7(2):75-81.

16. Unlu K, Aksunger A, Soker S, Ertem M. Mitomycin C primary trabeculectomy with releasable sutures in primary glaucoma. Jpn J Ophthalmol 2000;44:524-9.

17. Burchfield JC, Kolker AE, Cook SG. Endophthalmitis following trabeculectomy with releasable sutures. Arch Ophthalmol 1996;114:766.

18. Rosenberg LF, Siegfried CJ. Endophthalmitis following trabeculectomy with releasable sutures. Arch Ophthalmol 1996;114:767.

19. Jacob P, Thomas R, Mahajan A, et al. Releasable suture technique for trabeculectomy. Indian J Ophthalmol 1993;41(2):81-2.

20. Wanner J, Katz LJ. An Illustrative Review of Releasable Suture Techniques. Ophthalmic Surgery, Lasers and Imaging 2004; 35:465-474

Question 52

How should a postoperative bleb leak be managed?

Richard P. Mills

Early postoperative bleb leaks, appearing within the first two weeks, are managed differently than those appearing later in the postoperative period. The prognosis for long-term success of filtration is definitely impaired if an early postoperative leak is present. The Flurouracil Filtration Study showed at 1 year (5 years), the success rate for the 5-FU group was 80% (54%) in eyes without a leak, and 60% (28%) in those with a leak (p = .018).[1] Early leaks are easier to avoid intraoperatively than to manage postoperatively. This is particularly important if an antifibrotic agent such as mitomycin or 5-FU is employed. Closure of Tenon's capsule and conjunctiva in separate layers helps to tamponade the internal surface of the conjunctival wound. Use of a taper-point rather than cutting needle and 9-0 or 10-0 suture creates a needle track that is more easily plugged by the suture material. Testing of the wound with fluorescein after inflation of the bleb through the paracentesis helps to identify areas that need tighter closure.

Early leaks due to conjunctival buttonhole are best resutured when discovered using a mattress, figure-of-8, or purse-string suture on a taper-point needle. If the early leak is at the wound edge, most will seal spontaneously. Topical steroid should be reduced or eliminated, and short-acting topical or systemic inhibitors of aqueous production such as dorzolamide or diamox given to reduce the flow through the leak. As soon as the Seidel test becomes negative, the aqueous flow inhibitors should be stopped and the steroids given frequently. If the leak does not seal within 10-14 days, it should be sutured (see above).

A late leak may heal spontaneously, especially if it is the first leak, if it developed following some kind of trauma, or if it is slow. Antibiotic prophylaxis

247

may be useful, but should not be continued chronically.[2] Suturing is seldom effective because of the thinness and rigidity of the conjunctiva. Definitive treatment is indicated soon if the anterior chamber is shallowed or flat, or if there is hypotony maculopathy. Because there is a 25 times relative risk for endophthalmitis in the presence of bleb leak, chronic leaks should probably be repaired.[3] Mechanical, thermal, and chemical treatments for late leak have all been advocated, but if the leak is a product of a very thin bleb, surgical revision is the best option.[4]

Most surgeons advocate conjunctival advancement since it has a good track record of preserving bleb function.[5,6] Viscoelastic is placed intracamerally and the eye rotated downward using a clear corneal traction suture. The conjunctiva is incised posterior and lateral to the thin, ischemic bleb, which is either excised or denuded of epithelium Excision allows the underlying scleral flap to be resutured or reinforced. "Wing" peritomy incisions on either side of the bleb should be generous. Sharp and blunt dissection of all posterior adhesions of conjunctiva and Tenon's to sclera is essential to advancement of the flap to the limbus. Occasionally, a relaxing incision of conjunctiva in the fornix is necessary to release tension on the flap (this is surprisingly easy to close at the end of the operation). The flap is sutured at the "wings" with a taut anterior edge in a position with the least posterior traction. Additional suture is placed to ensure a watertight closure; if necessary a partial thickness keratotomy groove just anterior to the limbus provides a good anchor for suture.

In the event that insufficient conjunctiva is available locally for an advancement flap, an autograft 50% larger than the area to be covered can be harvested from inferiorly or from the fellow eye. Orientatation of the limbal edge should be maintained to preserve stem cell function. Meticulous suturing is necessary, and early leaks are common.[7] Similarly, if the original scleral flap is atrophic or necrotic, reinforcement with eye bank sclera or preserved pericardium cut freehand to overlie the edges of the defect can be sutured at the corners using 8-0 vicryl or similar suture.

REFERENCES

1. Parrish RK II, Schiffman JC, Feuer WJ, Heuer DK, Fluorouracil Filtering Surgery Study Group. Prognosis and risk factors for early postoperative wound leaks after trabeculectomy with and without 5-fluorouracil. Am J Ophthalmol, 2001; 132:633-40.

2. Wand M, Quintillani R, Robinson A. Antibiotic prophylaxis in eyes with filtration blebs: survey of glaucoma specialists, microbiological study and recommendations. J Glaucoma, 1995;104:816-822.

3. Soltau JB, Rothman RF, Budenz DL, Greenfield DS, Feuer W, Liebmann JM, Ritch R. Risk factors for glaucoma filtering bleb infections. Arch Ophthalmol, 2000;118:338-42.

4. Burnstein AL, WuDunn D, Knotts SL, Catoira Y, Cantor LB. Conjunctival advancement versus nonincisional treatment for late-onset glaucoma filtering bleb leaks. Ophthalmology, 2002;109:71-5.

5. Budenz DL, Chen PP, Weaver YK. Conjunctival advancement for late-onset filtering bleb leaks: indications and outcomes. Arch Ophthalmol, 1999;117:1014-9.

6. Wadhwani RA, Bellows AR, Hutchinson BT. Surgical repair of leaking filtering blebs. Ophthalmology, 2000;107:1681-7.

7. Schnyder CC, Shaarawy T, Ravinet E, Achache F, Uffer S, Mermoud A. Free conjunctival autologous graft for bleb repair and bleb reduction after trabeculectomy and nonpenetrating filtering surgery. J Glaucoma, 2002;11:10-6.

Question 53

When should a choroidal effusion after trabeculectomy be drained?

Neeru Gupta

Fluid accumulation in the suprachoroidal space may occur following trabeculectomy. Clinically, fundus examination typically reveals darkness of the uvea with the characteristic quadri- lobed appearance, corresponding to the firm attachments of the choroid to the vortex vein ampullae. Occasionally, the effusions may appear annular or flat. A B-scan ultrasound can help distinguish this from a retinal detachment by the acute anterior angle and its extension to the ora serrata.

Low intraocular pressure in the post-operative period following trabeculectomy can lead to choroidal effusions. In most cases, these resolve either spontaneously, or with conservative medical therapy. Anterior chamber shallowing and some degree of inflammation are often seen. Effective medical therapy typically involves cycloplegic-mydriatic drop, topical steroid and may include osmotic agents.

Choroidal effusions that are persistent, can lead to prolonged structural abnormalities, and threaten ocular function. Surgical drainage of these effusions is indicated as a last effort to prevent major complications. A flat anterior chamber with lens-cornea touch is an indication for surgical intervention as soon as possible. Progressive shallowing of the anterior chamber with forward displacement of the lens-iris diaphragm carries the risks of pupillary block, peripheral anterior synechiae, secondary glaucoma, cataract and corneal edema. If no clinical improvement is noted despite medical therapy for several days, drainage of the suprachoroidal space should be considered. A flat anterior chamber with inflammation and a failing bleb, is an additional indication to intervene surgically, and may well rescue the filtering site. Apposition of retinal tissue to the posterior lens surface or implant, or persistent apposition of retinal tissue to itself "choroidal kissing", may lead to permanent adhesions and retinal detachment, and should also be considered for drainage.

The drainage site should be selected at the site of maximal fluid accumulation. A scleral incision is placed 6mm to 8mm behind the limbus, and suprachoroidal fluid released slowly. This usually deepens the anterior chamber, and reformation of the anterior chamber can also be performed. Following trabeculectomy, in the presence of progressive ocular compromise, draining choroidal effusions can restore normal ocular relationships, minimize the complications of flat anterior chamber, and provide the best chance of preserving sight.

REFERENCES

1. Bellows AR. Chylack LT Jr., Hutchinson BT. Choroidal detachment. Ophthalmology, 88: 1107, 1981.

2. Berke SJ, Bellows RA, Shingleton BJ, Richter CU, Hutchinson BT. Chronic and recurrent choroidal detachment after glaucoma filtering surgery. Ophthalmology, 94: 154-162, 1987.

3. Brubaker RF, Pederson JE. Ciliochoroidal detachment. Survey of Ophthalmology, 27: 281-289, 1983.

4. Vela MA, Campbell DG. Hypotony and ciliochoroidal detachment following pharmacologic aqueous suppressant therapy in previously filtered patients. Ophthalmology, 92: 50-57, 1985.

Question 54

How should hypotony maculopathy due to overfiltration be managed ?

Robert L. Stamper

While modern filtering surgery is quite successful, several complications may follow even the most expertly done case. Hypotony occurs in about 10% of cases in the early postoperative period associated usually with over filtration. It may be even more common when antifibrotic agents such as mitomycin-C (MMC) or 5-fluorouracil (5-FU) are used. Most of the time hypotony is transient and improves within a few days or weeks of surgery. If hypotony persists, structural changes can occur in the eye. Some of the problems that are caused or exacerbated by hypotony include serous choroidal detachments, cataract, corneal edema, visual distortion and a peculiar chorio-retinal condition called hypotony maculopathy.

Hypotony Maculopathy occurs in about 4% (1.3-7%) of filtering operations with MMC or 5-FU. In this condition, the sclera and choroid are thrown into small folds at the back of the eye which cause significant visual disturbance. The pathophysiology seems to be the collapse of the posterior sclera causing the folds. The loss of vision is usually gradual after the hypotony has persisted for a month or more. The condition is recognized by characteristic striae or folds in the macular area which do not leak or stain with flourescein. (Fig. 1) Young Caucasian myopes having their first filtering surgery seem to be at greatest risk. The condition is likely to be bilateral if hypotony occurs in the second eye. Most cases are reversible, even if present for many months, if the hypotony is reversed. Therefore, the management of the maculopathy is essentially the management of the hypotony.

The first approach is to identify the cause of the hypotony. Hypotony after filtration surgery may be caused by overfiltration (most common), a leaking

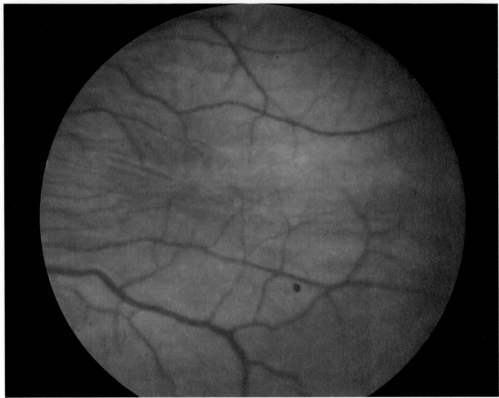

Figure 1. Hypotony maculopathy. Note striae in macula.

bleb, an inadvertent cyclodialysis cleft or persistent choroidal detachment (may be cause or effect). A leaking bleb is beyond the scope of this chapter.

In the early postoperative period, atropine should be utilized to facilitate aqueous production and to facilitate closure of a cyclodialysis cleft if present. Rapid tapering of steroid use is recommended to also facilitate the episcleral healing of the filtering site. Pressure on the bleb site with an oversize bandage contact lens, torpedo pressure patch, compression sutures or Simmons shell all have their advocates although in my hands, the compression sutures work the best for overfiltration in the early postoperative period. These sutures (8 or 9-0 nylon) are placed from cornea anteriorly to Tenon's capsule posterior to the bleb at each side of the bleb about 1 cm apart often help to delimit the bleb and prevent fluid from tracking inferiorly. Compression sutures can also be combined with some form of irritation of the bleb to encourage fibrosis.

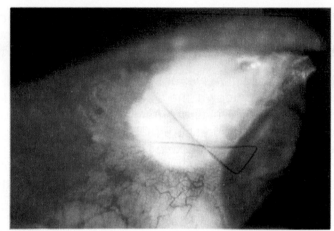

Figure 2. Compression suture at one end of bleb from cornea to Tenon's capsule (NOT epis-clera) .

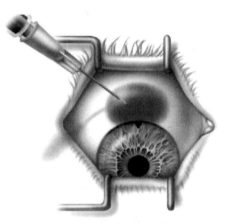

Figure 3. Blood patch. Autologous blood injection into filtering bleb. Adapted from Stamper, Lieberman and Drake: Becker-Shaffer's Diagnosis and Therapy of the Glaucomas, Seventh Edition. 1999, St. Louis, Mosby

The traditional irritants such as cryoapplication, diathermy or topical chemicals are not effective if MMC or 5-FU have been used. Autologous blood, injected into the bleb, has been useful although it may have to be repeated two or three times before results are seen. One or two cc of blood is withdrawn from the antecubital vein using a 19g needle. The needle is then switched to 25g 5/8 inch (1.5cm) and about 0.5 ml of blood is injected into the bleb from a site about 1 cm temporal. This all must be done quite rapidly before the blood clots. Occasionally some blood tracks into the anterior chamber but this usually clears within 24 hours. The process can be repeated in a month if there is little or no effect from the first one.

Finally, if the more conservative approaches fail, surgical revision is indicated. The bleb is taken down, the scleral flap is resutured and the bleb is resected and resutured. Palmberg has advocated total closure of the scleral flap so that intraocular pressure (IOP) rises to 25 mm Hg in the early postoperative period as an effective method to rapidly reverse the maculopathy. Later the sutures can be lysed with argon laser to control the IOP. However, if IOP is restored to 10 mm Hg or more, with a little patience, the maculopathy slowly reverses and vision usually recovers.

Question 55

What are the risk factors for bleb-related endophthalmitis?

Henry Jampel

Bleb-related endophthalmitis has been increasing recognized over the past decade as a serious, and all too common, complication of trabeculectomy. I am concerned enough about bleb-related endophthalmitis that I mention the possibility to all patients as part of the informed consent before surgery. I try to remind all my patients with filtration blebs on every visit that if they notice any symptoms or signs of possible ocular infection that they contact my office immediately. Other colleagues of mine hand their patients a wallet-sized card with the signs and symptoms and a phone number to contact.

A reduction in the occurrence of bleb-related endophthalmitis might be achieved through knowledge of the risk factors for bleb-related endophthalmitis and modification of those risks factors that can be altered. Identification of risk factors is classically performed through case-control studies, in which persons with a condition or disease (cases) are compared with persons without the condition or disease (controls) with regard to various personal characteristics and exposures. For bleb-related endophthalmitis, one would compare patients with filtration operations and endophthalmitis to patients with filtration operations without endophthalmitis.

Two recent case-control studies[1,2], one performed by our group, provide what is in my opinion the most current and definitive information available about the risk factors for bleb related endophthalmitis. A synthesis of the results of these two studies can be most easily understood by dividing risk factors into three groups: pre-operative, including patient characteristics, intraoperative, and post-operative (table). We found no patient or preoperative characteristics that were risk factors, although Soltau et al. found that younger age and black race were risk factors. In terms of operative risk factors, both studies found that blebs placed inferiorly were at higher risk for infection. We included full-thickness procedures in our analysis, and found them to be a risk factor as well. In our study, intraoperative use of mitomycin C was a risk factor, and combined cataract and glaucoma surgery was protective against infection. All of the patients in the study of Soltau et al. had received an antifibrosis agent and the authors matched for type of surgery (trabeculectomy alone or combined with cataract surgery, so those risk factors could not be analyzed in their study.

The postoperative risk factor stressed in the paper of Soltau et al. was bleb leak. The odds of an infected eye having a bleb leak at the time of diagnosis was 26 times greater than a non-infected eye having a bleb leak at any time postoperatively. One can infer that prompt diagnosis of bleb leaks and treatment of the leak might reduce the risk of bleb infection. Our most provocative result concerning postoperative risk factors was that the use of antibiotics either episodically, but especially chronically, was associated with an increased risk of infection (Odds ratio of 2.10 (1.09-4.02) and 5.94 (2.09-16.9), for episodic and chronic use, respectively). This finding should make glaucoma surgeons think twice about prescribing antibiotics chronically after surgery to prevent infection.

I believe that the "take home" messages from these two studies are to be cautious with the use of mitomycin C, think carefully about the use of routine chronic antibiotics to prevent bleb infection, and to increase one's level of alertness, and perhaps intervene surgically, at the sight of a bleb leak.

Table 1. Risk factors for bleb-related infection

Patient and preoperative characteristics	
	Younger age ?
	Black race ?
Surgical characteristics	
	Full-thickness procedures
	Glaucoma operation without cataract surgery
	Inferiorly placed bleb
	Intraoperative mitomycin C
Postoperative characteristics	
	Bleb leak
	Episodic or chronic antibiotic use

REFERENCES

1. Jampel HD, Quigley HA, Kerrigan-Baumrind LA, Melia BM, Friedman D, Barron Y. Risk factors for late-onset infection following glaucoma filtration surgery. Arch Ophthalmol, 2001.Jul.;119.(7.):1001.-8., 119: 1001-1008.

2. Soltau JB, Rothman RF, Budenz DL et al. Risk factors for glaucoma filtering bleb infections. Arch Ophthalmol, 2000.Mar.;118.(3.):338.-42., 118: 338-342.

Question 56

How is a failing bleb diagnosed and managed?

Hitching Roger A.

The term 'failing bleb' can be reserved for those eyes where the intraocular pressure (IOP) either, a) after surgery never settles at a predetermined Target IOP, or b) at a later stage increases above the steady state achieved post filtration surgery. It is the purpose of this article to discuss a), as this problem is one of the commonest problems adversely affecting successful surgical outcomes in glaucoma today.

The failure of the IOP to settle at the predetermined Target level follows a series of 'inflammatory' changes around the operation site whereby activated fibroblasts secrete collagen. This process leads to increased resistance to aqueous absorption by the capillaries in Tenons capsule and the conjunctiva. To first diagnose the 'failing bleb' it is important to recognise stages in the development of a 'successful' bleb

Development of the 'successful' bleb

After glaucoma surgery the dissected conjunctiva becomes oedematous showing as tissue swelling without hyperaemia. This is soon to be replaced by localised tissue elevation from the presence of aqueous percolating through the superficial scleral flap. With the passage of time this elevation subsides leaving only an appearance ranging from a translucent elevation to a flattened area of conjunctiva overlying the scleral flap. All these stages are associated with an IOP in the mid 'teens with a small diurnal fluctuation.

Diagnosis of the 'failing' bleb

The inflammatory changes preventing this sequence of events produce local tissue swelling with hyperaemia centred on the operation site. At this stage the site is becoming populated with activated fibroblasts, either converted from 'inactive' cells pre-existing at the site, or chemotactically attracted from adjacent areas. This is followed by localised disruption in the otherwise smooth course of the conjunctival vessels ('corkscrew changes') due to contraction of newly secreted collagen. Left untreated this process concludes with gross conjunctival contraction. The conjunctiva contracts towards a collagen anchor, with fornix based flaps this is at the limbus, with limbal based flaps it is towards the forniceal conjunctival incision. By this time the operation can be said to have failed; the patient will be worse off than before because the operation site will now be populated with 'activated' fibroblasts, and these will respond more vigorously to reoperation than for the initial procedure.

It should be noted that these signs can occur quite independently of increasing IOP, especially when associated with choroidal effusions- where the IOP can be misleadingly low, although the process concludes with an IOP often significantly higher than preoperatively.

Management

As the period between surgery and irretrievable wound healing is short, and may be no more than 2 weeks, it is imperative to recognise the signs of impending failure and mitigate them as far as possible. The methods available are divided into *Prevention* and *Treatment*. Prevention is to recognise those eyes likely to have:

1) Abnormal cell population in the conjunctiva-producing a heightened fibroblast response. Causes for this are listed below:

Coexisting conjunctival inflammatory disease

Blepharitis

Conjunctival inflammatory disease (Vernal)

Chronic glaucoma (and other topical) treatments

Previous conjunctival surgery

2) Coexisting ocular disease with abnormal blood aqueous barrier, where the aqueous stimulates a heightened fibroblast response

  Chronic uveitis/Scleritis

  Previous intraocular surgery

3) Demographic preconditions leading to heightened fibroblast response

  Youth

  'Black races'

Conditions under 1) above can be pre-treated with 1 month of a topical steroid. The writer uses the mineralocorticoid Fluoromethalone (FML) 3-4 times a day for this purpose. Additionally any topically applied medication that could be causing the inflammation should be withdrawn.

Conditions under 2) above can be pre-treated with a topical steroid, here a glucocorticoid such as Dexamethzone 0.1% 3-4 times a day will usually suffice.

The enhanced inflammatory response can be suppressed with a per-or post operative antimetabolite. In order of potency: topical beta irradiation< preoperative 5 fluorouracil (25ug/ml*5 mins) < peroperative mitomycin (0.2<0.4ug/ml*2-4 mins).

The signs of inflammation and scarring noted above may be suppressed with the same approaches. Intensive topical steroids will reverse the signs of conjunctival hyperaemia. However this time it will need to be a glucocorticoid such as Dexamethazone 0.1%. This treatment will need to be augmented with postoperative injections of 5 fluorouracil (25ug/ml/0.2ml) around the operation site (but not into the drainage area itself, because of the risk of 5 FU entering the eye, where being a highly alkaline solution it is toxic to the corneal endothelium). It should be noted that these treatments will have little effect once the stage of 'corkscrew vessels' has developed.

Additionally procedures designed to enhance the egress of aqueous can help in the stage of inflammation. Removal of a (the) releasable suture will facilitate aqueous egress (resistance around the loop will also identify a site of fibrous tissue deposition). 'Needling' of the bleb (a procedure designed to incise fibrous tissue sheets that can develop over the superficial scleral flap and/or 'encysting' the aqueous in the subconjunctival space) will promote the exit of aqueous again.

To date the procedures for managing the postoperative wound healing response are less than perfect. This is partly because we do not have a method for assessing the height of the response and partly because the science of wound healing suppression is still in its infancy. The procedures outlined above will however ensure a better outcome than had been hitherto possible.

Which patients are at most risk for post-operative vision loss following trabeculectomy?

Andrew C. Crichton

Further visual damage as a result of surgery is one of the greatest concerns of the glaucoma surgeon. This is especially the case in situations of threatened fixation where there is no margin for further loss. The questions we must ask ourselves in preparation for surgery are firstly, how great is the risk and secondly, what can we do about it?

The literature would suggest that we have a justification for being concerned but fortunately the risk is small. For the purpose of this discussion, I acknowledge that references to "wipeout" are certainly present prior to 1993, but I have selected to limit the review to more recent publications in recognition or our more advanced refinements with surgical techniques.

An extensive review from 1993 by Costa of 508 eyes showed 4 eyes suffering from loss of central vision[1]. Although this figure represents less than 1%, when the data was isolated to look at patients with markedly damaged fields, the incidence of loss was actually higher at 3.28%. The mean age of the patients was higher in this group and severe post-operative hypotony appeared to be a risk. Levene in 1992 reviewed 96 eyes with severe visual field loss finding 1 patient suffering further damage to less than 20/200[2]. 408 patients were also reported by Thiel in 2000 finding that 0.5% suffered loss of fixation immediately after surgery[3].

Reassuringly however, we have some evidence to suggest that the risk of loss may be even less. Martinez in 1993 reviewed 31 patients with split fixation and found no individuals suffering from further loss[4]. More recently in 1996, Grunewald reviewed 50 eyes again without finding any wipeout[5].

All the previous studies involved traditional surgery (trabeculectomy) including the occasional valve but it is also worth mentioning a study by Ates in 1999 citing 54 eyes with advanced field loss receiving deep sclerectomy and collagen implant[6]. No patients suffered loss of vision.

Fortunately the magnitude of the problem is not large but for the rare individual the situation is obviously calamitous. We must therefore direct our efforts to eliminate the wipeout in these few patients.

Obviously understanding the etiology of the problem clearly would allow the surgeon to minimize risk but with so few patients affected, any definitive answer is surely beyond our reach. We do have suggestions by Costa that age and hypotony may be risks. We could speculate that a marked, sudden decompression could cause damage to the circulation or nerve fibers at the lamina cribosa. Additionally there could be edema associated with hypotony that may cause similar compression and damage. In the same article there was acknowledgement of visual loss in 2 patients with pressure spikes and the recognition that early post-operative spikes may go unrecognized. Another concern worth mentioning is the potential risk of local anaesthetic, primarily retro-bulbar. One must always acknowledge that there may be a risk to the optic nerve with pressure in the cone.

Ultimately then we must ask ourselves how surgically we can minimize the risk for the patient and decrease the possibility of wipeout even more. Complicating our efforts, however, is the more recent awareness of the need for very low target pressures with severe visual field loss and the further requirement for technique modification.

Our goal for surgery for all individuals, but especially for these patients, is to avoid hypotony and intraocular pressure spikes. The requirements, therefore, for trabeculectomy are an efficient, meticulous technique. Considerations could include: minimizing anterior chamber collapse with a continuous infusion, adjustable sutures, and of course, an evaluation of the pressure at the end of the procedure. To obtain the low IOP an anti-metabolite such as Mitomycin or 5-Flourourcil would likely be required.

Post-operatively, Diamox can be used overnight to blunt any potential pressure spike and certainly IOP can be checked sooner that 24 hours.

Perhaps in a perfect world we may evolve to a technique involving deep sclerectomy under topical anaesthetic[6], stripping of the canal of Schlemm, use of a potentially safer anti-metabolite[7], and goniopuncture when appropriate to increase flow by creating a full thickness procedure. One could think of this as an "ultra-guarded filtration".

Study	Number of Patients	Loss of Fixation
1992 Levene	96	0.5%
1993 Costa	508	3.28%
2000 Thiel	408	0.5%
1997 Martinez	31	0%
1996 Grunewald	50	0%
1999 Ates	54	0%

REFERENCES

1. Costa VP, Smith M, Spaeth GL, Gandham S, Markovitz B. Loss of visual acuity after trabeculectomy. Ophthalmol, 1993;100(5):599-612.

2. Levene RZ. Central visual field, visual acuity, and sudden visual loss after glaucoma surgery. Ophthalmic Surg, 1992;23(6):388-94.

3. Thiel HJ, Denk PO, Knorr M. Are filtering interventions in glaucoma patients with extensive visual field defects associated with higher functional risk? Ophthalmologe, 2000;97(5):336-41.

4. Martinez JA, Brown RH, Lynch MG, Caplan MB. Risk of postoperative visual loss in advanced glaucoma. Am J Ophthalmol, 1993;115(3):332-37.

5. Grunewald F, Bresson-Dumont, Bechetoille A. Is trabeculectomy without danger incase of threatened fixation? J Fr Ophthalmol, 1996;19(4):253-8.

6. Ates H, Andac K, Uretmen O. Non-penetrating deep slcerectomy and collagen implant surgery in glaucoma patients with advanced field loss. Int Ophthalmol, 1999; 23(3):123-8.

7. Mead AL, Wong TTL, Cordeiro MF, Anderson IK, Khaw PT. Evaluation of anti-TGF-β2 antibody as a new postoperative anti-searring agent in glaucoma surgery. Invest Ophthalmol Vis Sci, 2003;44:3394-3401.

Question 58

What are the indications for combined procedures (cataract and glaucoma)

Lili Farrokh-Siar

Michelle Colev

Ahmad A. Aref

Theodore Krupin

The debate about surgical management of coexisting cataract in patients with primary open-angle glaucoma (POAG) is ongoing and has changed in the past two decades in response to development of phacoemulcification, intraocular lens implantation, and new filtration procedures. Ophthalmologists have been interested in combined operations since Birge's description of cataract extraction with iridencleisis in 1952.[1] In theory there are at least three potential advantages for the combined procedure: 1) long-term control of intraocular pressure (IOP) and removal of the visual impairment with one procedure, 2) reduction of a transient pressure spike in the initial postoperative period[2] that may be critical in patients with advanced POAG, and 3) patient convenience because two procedures are done during a single operation.

Sequential management of cataract and glaucoma (Figure 1)

The ultimate surgical goals for POAG patients with coexisting cataract should be adequate IOP control and enhanced quality of life by improving vision and decreasing IOP-lowering medications. The trend in the

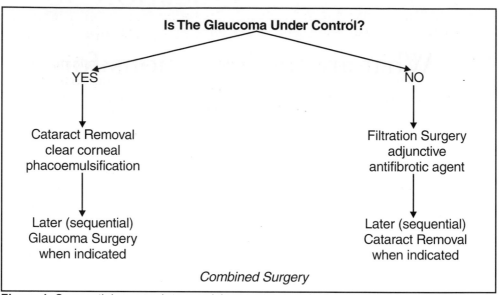

Figure 1. Sequential approach to coexisitng cataract and primary open-angle glaucoma.

mid-1900's to perform combined surgery has shifted to staged (sequential) surgeries based on a number of publications and clinical observations:

- Combined surgery risks more intraoperative and postoperative complications than either cataract extraction or trabeculectomy alone.

- Visual recovery is faster when cataract removal is performed by itself than when it is combined with trabeculectomy.

- Cataract removal alone in an eye with stable POAG usually has a beneficial effect on postoperative pressure control: IOP is equal or lower on the same or fewer medications.[3]

- Glaucoma control after cataract removal alone avoids complications associated with an unneeded antifibrotic filtration bleb.

- Cataract removal via temporal clear cornea phacoemulsification results in the quickest visual recovery and avoids superior manipulation of the conjunctiva and limbal tissues, preserving superior conjunctiva if a trabeculectomy is needed.

- Trabeculectomy alone with adjunctive 5-fluorouracil (5FU)[4] or mitomycin-c (MMC)[5] results in a better filtration bleb and lower IOP than a combined procedure with either of these antifibrotic agents.

- Initial antifibrotic trabeculectomy is equally effective in a temporal clear corneal incision pseudophakic eye as a phakic eye.

- Cataract removal in an eye with a functioning bleb has minimal effect on long-term bleb survival.[6, 7] Chen et al[7] showed that 95% of eyes with a functioning bleb that underwent phacoemulsification did not require further glaucoma surgery during an 18-month period.

A recent meta-analysis by Hylton et al[8] has confirmed the widely known association of accelerated progression of cataract following filtration surgery. Possible mechanisms for this occurrence include alterations of the rate of aqueous humor production or its composition, toxicity from antifibrotic agents, and/or postoperative inflammation or shallowing of the anterior chamber. We do not believe this association should lead to performing combined surgery at the time of trabeculectomy if the patient's cataract is not visually significant, just as we do not believe combined surgery should be performed at the time of cataract surgery if the patient's glaucoma is stable. A sequential approach to eyes with coexisting POAG and cataract has the advantage of individual application of each step; temporal corneal phacoemulcification with its technical precision and rapid visual recovery, and superior antifibrotic trabeculectomy with its high success rate in phakic and pseudophakic eyes. In most cases, a sequential approach is more prudent than performing combined surgery. This staged approach maximizes benefits while minimizing complications.

Indications for combined surgery

The decision to perform a combined procedure needs to be individualized in patients with both cataract and POAG. Some patients may not be able to tolerate the two anesthesias, longer recovery period, or cost required for staged procedures (e.g., general medical health, distance from ophthalmology care, or social status). Patients with both uncontrolled and advanced glaucoma, and a visually handicapping cataract could benefit from a combined procedure. While cataract removal alone has a positive benefit on IOP control, it is not a substitute for trabeculectomy.

Our approach to combined surgery is a two-site procedure: temporal clear corneal phacoemulsification and a superior MMC trabeculectomy (Figure 2).

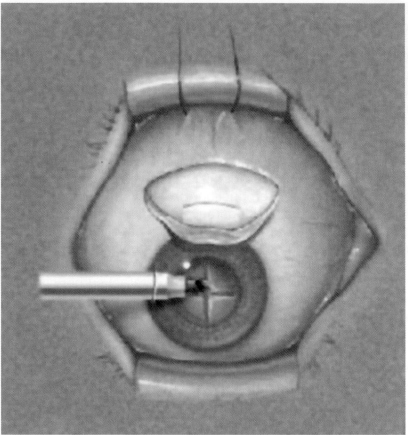

Figure 2. Two-site combined cataract and trabeculectomy. Superior limbus-based antifibrotic trabeculectomy and temporal clear corneal phacoemulcification removal of cataract with posterior chamber lens implant.

- Tezel et al[9] reported better IOP control, reduced requirement for glaucoma medications, and a lower complication rate with phacotrabeculectomy than ECCE-trabeculectomy.

- 5-FU is not as effective as MMC during combined surgery.[10, 11] Also, both of these antifibrotic agents are less effective in combined surgery compared to trabeculectomy alone.

- The two-site approach with MMC has a weak advantage (less need for postoperative medications) than the one-site approach.[11, 12] This may be explained by the fact that the two-site approach reduces conjunctival manipulation inflammation at the trabeculectomy site.

- The type of intraocular lens does not have any effect on the outcome of the glaucoma procedure and intraocular pressure.[13]

Summary

A sequential rather than the combined approach is a safer and more useful option in most open-angle glaucoma patients with coexisting cataract. Combined surgery may be indicated in cases where a patient suffers *significant* visual handicap due to cataracts as well as uncontrolled glaucoma. The combined procedure may also be indicated based on cost, medical, or social patient issues.

REFERENCES

1. Birge HL. Glaucoma with cataract surgically cured in single operation. Trans Am Ophthalmol Soc, 1952;50:241-63.

2. Krupin T, Feitl ME, Bishop KI. Postoperative intraocular pressure rise in open-angle glaucoma patients after cataract or combined cataract-filtration surgery. Ophthalmology, 1989;96:579-84.

3. Shingleton BJ, Gamell LS, O'Donoghue MW, et al. Long-term changes in intraocular pressure after clear corneal phacoemulsification: normal patients versus glaucoma suspect and glaucoma patients. J Cataract Refract Surg, 1999;25:885-90.

4. Park HJ, Weitzman M, Caprioli J. Temporal corneal phacoemulsification combined with superior trabeculectomy. A retrospective case-control study. Arch Ophthalmol, 1997; 115:318-23.

5. Derick RJ, Evans J, Baker ND. Combined phacoemulsification and trabeculectomy versus trabeculectomy alone: a comparison study using mitomycin-C. Ophthalmic Surg Lasers, 1998;29:707-13.

6. Caprioli J, Park HJ, Kwon YH, et al. Temporal corneal phacoemulsification in filtered glaucoma patients. Trans Am Ophthalmol Soc, 1997;95:153-67.

7. Chen PP, Weaver YK, Budenz DL, et al. Trabeculectomy function after cataract extraction. Ophthalmology, 1998;105:1928-35.

8. Hylton C, Congdon N, Friedman D, et al. Cataract after glaucoma filtration surgery. Am J Ophthalmol, 2003;135:231-2.

9. Tezel G, Kolker AE, Kass MA, et al. Comparative results of combined procedures for glaucoma and cataract: II. Limbus-based versus fornix-based conjunctival flaps. Ophthalmic Surg Lasers, 1997;28:551-7.

10. Wong PC, Ruderman JM, Krupin T, et al. 5-Fluorouracil after primary combined filtration surgery. Am J Ophthalmol, 1994;117:149-54.

11. Jampel HD, Friedman DS, Lubomski LH, et al. Effect of technique on intraocular pressure after combined cataract and glaucoma surgery: An evidence-based review. Ophthalmology, 2002;109:2215-24.

12. Wyse T, Meyer M, Ruderman JM, et al. Combined trabeculectomy and phacoemulsification: a one-site vs a two-site approach. Am J Ophthalmol, 1998;125:334-9.

13. Casson RJ, Salmon JF. Combined surgery in the treatment of patients with cataract and primary open-angle glaucoma. J Cataract Refract Surg, 2001;27:1854-63.

Question 59

What indications are there for non penetrating surgery

Roberto G. Carassa

In recent years non-penetrating surgery achieved great interest as a possible alternative to trabeculectomy. This class of procedures are mainly represented by *"deep sclerectomy"* and by *"viscocanalostomy"*. Similarly, both procedures are aimed at allowing drainage of the aqueous humor from the anterior chamber not through a patent scleral opening, but by slow percolation through the inner trabecular meshwork and/or Descemet membrane ("trabeculo-descemetic membrane"). This avoids sudden IOP drops, hypotonyies and flat chambers. The absence of anterior chamber opening and iridectomy limits the risk of cataract and infection. Compared to deep sclerectomy, viscocanalostomy is a step forward. In fact, this procedure is aimed not only at taking the advantages of being non-penetrating, as deep sclerectomy, but, most important, in restoring the physiological outflow pathway, thus avoiding any external filtration.[1] The indications for the 2 procedures are thus slightly different.

Deep sclerectomy

The surgical technique varies: generally, a 5x5-mm parabolic superficial flap, approximately 1/3 of scleral thickness is dissected. Some Authors, at this stage, in all or in selected cases only, apply a sponge soaked with Mitomicin C over the sclera in order to increase the success rate. A limbus-based triangle of deep sclera is then dissected as deep as to leave a thin layer of sclera over the choroid and the ciliary body. The dissection is carried anteriorly until Schlemm's canal is deroofed and 1-2 mm of Descemet's membrane are exposed. The inner flap is then removed, and, in order to avoid post-operative scarring, different implants are often used. The superficial scleral flap is then repositioned and sutured with two 10-0 nylon sutures. Finally, the conjunctiva is tightly closed.

Results show that the mean final IOP without adjunctive therapy is in the mid- high-teens, while the achievement of an IOP below 21 mmHg is obtained in 57-92%. It should be noted that up to 40% of the treated eyes undergo "trabeculo-descemet membrane" goniopuncture with Nd:YAG laser in the post-operative time.[2-4] When compared with trabeculectomy the success in achieving an IOP below 21 mmHg is comparable even though final IOPs are lower with trabeculectomy. The adjunctive use of Mitomicin C, increases the success rate and allows a better IOP control.[5] Complications are minor and fewer than those reported after trabeculectomy.

Deep sclerectomy has specific indications and contraindications, based on its intrinsic characteristics and on clinical results.

The procedure is not indicated in angle closure glaucomas, in neovascular glaucoma and in eyes with wide angle synechia or diffuse scarring of the conjunctiva in the surgical quadrant. As suggested by the Guidelines for Glaucoma of the European Glaucoma Society, deep sclerectomy is indicated in primary open angle glaucoma when target IOP is not very low. The advantages of being non-penetrating make the procedure particularly useful in aphakic eyes with vitreous in the anterior chamber, or in cases where a sudden drop in IOP should be avoided as in eyes with uncontrolled very high pressure or myopic eyes.

Viscocanalostomy

Different from deep sclerectomy, viscocanalostomy attempts to restore the impaired physiological aqueous outflow pathway allowing the aqueous to leave the eye not by simple external filtration but through Schlemm's canal and the episcleral veins. The procedure creates, in fact, a "chamber" inside the sclera which directly communicates both with Schlemm's canal and with the anterior chamber through the "trabeculo-descemetic membrane". A recent experimental study on mechanism of action showed the evidence of micro-openings throughout the wall of Schlemm's canal over 360 degrees which may be involved in the increased aqueous facility. [6]

The surgical technique of viscocanalostomy is characterized by 2 concentric scleral flaps. The outer flap, which will create the "roof" of the intra-scleral "chamber", is commonly dissected in a 5 x 5 mm parabolic shape, approximately 200μm deep. The inner scleral flap provides the access to Schlemm's canal and its removal leaves the space for the intrascleral chamber. A peculiar step in this procedure is the cannulation of Schlemm's canal and its slow filling with high molecular weight sodium hyaluronate which is obtained using a specific cannula Finally, the intrascleral "chamber" is tightly sealed by the outer scleral flap which is sutured back in place with 7 10-0 nylon stitches.

After viscocanalostomy the mean final IOPs range between 14 and 18 and an IOP below 21 mmHg is obtained in up to 76% of the cases. When compared to trabeculectomy, the latter allows a better IOP control with lower final pressures. Complications are minor and fewer than those reported after trabeculectomy. Filtering blebs are seldom seen and an external filtration can be detected in less than 30% of the cases.[7,8]

As for deep sclerectomy, viscocanalostomy has specific indications and contraindications. It cannot be effective when the angle is closed or neovascularized, or when Schlemm's canal is likely to be damaged. This is the case of previously operated eyes where an extensive cautery of the perilimbar area was made. Due to its final results the procedure is indicated in primary open angle glaucoma when target IOP is not very low (as indicated by the Guidelines for Glaucoma of the European Glaucoma Society). The advantage of the absence (or very reduced) external filtration make the technique safe and particularly indicated in eyes with chronic blepharitis, in lens contact wear or when surgery has to be performed in the lateral or inferior quadrants. Viscocanalostomy was shown effective also in uveitic glaucomas with well controlled inflammation.[9]

REFERENCES

1. Stegmann R, Pienaar A, Miller D: Viscocanalostomy for open-angle glaucoma in black african patients. J Cataract Refract Surg, 1999;25:316-322.

2. Mermoud A, Schnyder CC, Sickenberg M, Chiou AG, Hediguer SE, Faggioni R: Comparison of deep sclerectomy with collagen implant and trabeculectomy in open angle glaucoma. J Cataract Refract Surg, 1999;25:323-331.

3. Shaarawy T, Nguyen C, Schneyder C, Mermoud A: Comparative study between deep sclerectomy with and without collagen implant: long term follow up. Br J Ophthalmol, 2004;1:95-98.

4. Ambresin A, Shaarawy T, Mermoud A: Deep sclerectomy with collagen implant in one eye compared with trabeculectomy in the other eye of the same patient. J Glaucoma, 2002;11:214-220.

5. Kozobolis VP, Christodoulakis EV, Tzanakis N, Zacharopoulos I, Pallikaris IG: Primery deep sclerectomy with the use of mitomycin C in primary open-angle glaucoma. J Glaucoma, 2002;11:287-293.

6. Tamm ER, Carassa RG, Albert DM, Gabelt BT, Patel S, Rasmussen CA, Kaufman PL: Viscocanalostomy in Rhesus Monkeys. Arch Ophthalmol. 2004;122:1826-1838.

7. Shaarawy T, Nguyen C, Schneyder C, Mermoud A: Five year results of viscocanalostomy. Br J Ophthalmol, 2003;87:441-445.

8. Carassa RG, Bettin P, Fiori M, Brancato R: Viscocanalostomy versus Trabeculectomy in white adults affected by open-angle glaucoma: a 2-year randomized, controlled trial. Ophthalmology, 2003;110:882-887.

9. Miserocchi E, Carassa RG, Bettin P, Brancato R: Viscocanalostomy in patients with uveitis: a preliminary report. J Cataract and Refr Surg, 2004, 30:566-570.

Question 60

When should glaucoma drainage device be used in the surgical treatment of glaucoma?

Don Minckler

Pediatric glaucomas

Glaucoma drainage devices (GDDs) are good primary therapy for management of pediatric glaucomas associated with anterior segment anomalies or those following prior surgical or non-surgical trauma that preclude goniotomy or trabeculotomy. GDDs may be preferable to trabeculectomy in glaucoma-associated uveitis in children or adults, as their drainage function is more likely to survive recurring cycles of inflammation.[1] Anterior chamber tube placement is unwise if the chamber is shallow and cornea or lens tube-touch is likely. GDDs vary in size and shape and should only be used in children when orbital space and eye size are adequate.[2] GDDs have substantially less long-term risk of infection than trabeculectomy with antifibrotic agents, of particular importance in children. The principal long-term disadvantage of drainage devices in children is corneal endothelial decompensation.

Primary and secondary adult glaucomas

Adult glaucoma in pseudophakic eyes represents the largest group of candidates for GDDs. The most obvious indications for a GDD as the next step in surgical management of glaucoma include failure to achieve the desired target intraocular (IOP) range on maximal medical therapy, defined by the patient's tolerance and response to topical or systemic agents, and scarring of the conjunctiva superiorly. In most instances before GDDs are used, argon laser or selective laser trabeculoplasty will have already been done or not be possible because of angle-closure. Usually one or more trabeculectomies or other types of filtering surgery, with or without antifibrotic agents, will have failed.

GDDs seldom result in IOPs below the mid-teens, even with adjunctive topical or systemic medications. A relatively low target IOP range makes trabeculectomy the procedure of choice in most adult glaucomas, especially those with advanced visual field and optic nerve damage. Iridectomy is not necessary with GDDs, as they are relatively non-vulnerable to occlusion by iris.

Vitreous in the anterior chamber precludes successful use of a GDD as mobile vitreous will occlude the tube. Pars plana insertion of the drainage tube is preferred if the eye in question has undergone a complete vitrectomy as there is probably less risk of long-term corneal damage with pars plana placement of the tube. A pre-existing anterior chamber tube may be moved posteriorly and re-inserted via the pars plana if cataract surgery and or vitrectomy are subsequently performed. Pars plana tube insertion in phakic eyes is hazardous and likely to accelerate cataract formation, especially if there is tube-lens touch. Progressing peripheral anterior synechiae (PAS) may ratchet an anterior chamber tube forward and cause tube-cornea touch making insertion of an anterior chamber tube through PAS, when present, desirable. Anterior chamber tubes should protrude approximately 1.5 to 2 mm into the chamber to preclude sheathing and occlusion by extension of Decemet's membrane.[3]

Non valved pars plana or anterior chamber tubes (Baerveldt, Molteno) should always be inserted in two-stages utilizing two separate surgeries or internal or external temporary ligatures to prevent function for two-three weeks to enable pre- aqueous flow fibrous encapsulation of the explant.[3] A two-stage insertion, after explant encapsulation, is probably the safest method by which to minimize postoperative hypotony and choroidal hemorrhage in very high risk eyes. Pre-placement of a non-valved device (1st stage Baerveldt or Molteno) may provide desirable flexibility in cases where the necessity for a filtering procedure cannot be accurately predicted at the time of surgery (combined cataract & glaucoma surgery; pars plana vitrectomy; penetrating keratoplasty; complex retina-vitreous procedures).[4-9] GDDs increase the risk of graft rejection following penetrating keratoplasty.

Valved devices (Ahmed, Krupin) are inserted with the expectation of immediate postoperative function. However, there is some risk of hypotony due to leak around the tube at the insertion site or rarely "over filtration". Anterior chamber tubes should be inserted through full-thickness sclera for maximal stability.[3] Patch grafts of donor pericardium or sclera covering the anterior few millimeters of the tube reduce tube erosion and exposure and are technically easier than fashioning a host scleral flap.

The choice of GDD should be based on the surgeon's experience and expectations.[2,10,11] Non-valved GDDs provide desirable flexibility but require two-stage installation.[3] Specific contraindications for valved GDDs include high risks of bleeding or fibrin formation that may occlude the valve. De-valving occluded Ahmed valves weeks to months postoperatively may restore function. In any case, the valve is only useful until encapsulation occurs. Silicone oil in the vitreous and anterior chamber may percolate through valved tubes and excite subconjunctival inflammation, prevented if the explant is encapsulated before aqueous flow. The importance of explant surface area to successful IOP control has been well-demonstrated both clinically and experimentally.[7] A GDD can be fashioned from buckle materials and silicone rubber tubing (Schocket procedure) or a pre-existing encircling element (modified Schocket procedure) by connecting a segment of silicone tubing into the potential space between the buckle element and its capsule.[3, 12]

A recent randomized trial has reinforced the impression that mitomycin C applied during GDD installation does not enhance efficacy.[13]

REFERENCES

1. Hill RA, Heuer DK, Baerveldt G, Minckler DS, Martone JF: Molteno. Implantation for glaucoma in young patients. Ophthalmology, 1991;98:1042-1046.

2. Prata JA Jr, Mermoud A, LaBree L, and Minckler DS: In vitro and In vivo flow characteristics of glaucoma drainage implants. Ophthalmology, 1995;102:894-904.

3. Minckler DS: Glaucoma drainage devices, pathophysiology and surgical techniques. Ch 14. Glaucoma Surgical Techniques. Ophthalmology Monographs #4. American Academy of Ophthalmology, 1998.

4. McDonnell PJ, Robin JB, Schanzlin DJ, Minckler DS, Baerveldt G, Smith RE and Heuer D: Molteno implant for control of glaucoma in eyes after penetrating keratoplasty. Ophthalmology, 1988;95:364-369.

5. Lloyd MA, Heuer DK, 5. Baerveldt G, Minckler DS, Martone JF, Lean JS, and Liggett PE: Combined Molteno implantation and pars plana vitrectomy for neovascular glaucomas. Ophthalmology, 1991;98:1401-1405.

6. Lloyd MA, Sedlak T, Heuer DK, Minckler DS, Baerveldt G, Lee MB, Martone JF: Clinical experience with the single-plate Molteno implant in complicated glaucomas. Update of a pilot study. Ophthalmology, 1991;99:679-687.

7. Heuer DK, Lloyd MA, Abrams DA, Baerveldt G, Minckler DS, Lee MB, and Martone JF: Which is better? One or two? A randomized clinical trial of single-plate versus double-plate Molteno implantation for glaucomas in aphakia and pseudophakia. Ophthalmology, 1992;99:1512-1519.

8. Lloyd MA, Baerveldt G, Fellenbaum PS, Sidoti PA, Minckler DS, Martone FJ, LaBree L, and Heuer DK: Intermediate-term results of a randomized clinical trial of the 350 versus the 500-mm2 Baerveldt implant. Ophthalmology, 1994;101:1456-1464.

9. Varma R, Heuer DK, Lundy DC, Baerveldt G, Lee PP, and Minckler DS: Pars plana Baerveldt tube insertion with vitrectomy in glaucomas associated with pseudophakia and aphakia. Am J Ophthalmol, 1995;119:401-407.

10. Taglia DP, Perkins TW, Gangnon R, et al. Comparison of the Ahmed glaucoma Valve, the Krupin eye Valve with Disk, and the double-plate Molteno implant. J Glaucoma, 2002; 11(4):347-53.

11. Molteno AC, Bevin TH, Herbison P, Houliston MJ. Otago glaucoma surgery outcome study: long-term follow-up of cases of primary glaucoma with additional risk factors drained by Molteno implants. Ophthalmology, 2001;108:2193-200.

12. Sidoti PA, Minckler DS, Baerveldt G, Lee PP, and Heuer DK: Aqueous tube shunt to a pre-existing episcleral encircling element in the treatment of complicated glaucomas. Ophthalmology, 1994;101:1036-1043.

13. Costa VP, Azuara-Blanco A, Netland PA, Lesk MR, Arcieri ES. Efficacy and Safety of Adjunctive Mitomycin C during Ahmed Glaucoma Valve Implantation. Ophthalmology, 2004;111:1071-1076.

Question 61

Is mitomycin C or 5-Fluorouracil useful with aqueous shunting procedures?

Troy M. Tanji

Dale K. Heuer

Aqueous shunting surgery may be useful when a conventional glaucoma filtering procedure has failed or is unlikely to succeed. An aqueous shunt consists of a silicone tube connected to an equatorial explant(s), the size and shape of which, as well as presence or absence of valve on which, vary among the commercially available devices. The tube is inserted into the eye to allow aqueous flow to the bleb surrounding the equatorial plate, from which the aqueous passively diffuses into the surrounding fibrous capsule.

Clinical studies have reported early success rates of 25% to 100% in a variety of glaucomas. Larger surface-area explants, such as the double-plate Molteno implant, tend to give lower intraocular pressures (IOPs).[1] However, an upper limit apparently exists, as explants with even greater surface areas did not result in lower IOPs.[2] Long-term results of aqueous shunts have also shown a gradual decline in IOP control over time, which has been attributed (at least in part) to increased capsular fibrosis around the equatorial explant.[3] Wound-healing modulation with agents, such as 5-fluorouracil (5-FU) and mitomycin C (MMC), increases the success rate of conventional glaucoma filtering surgery, raising the question of whether such an approach might also be helpful in aqueous shunting procedures.

Whiteside-Michel and Egbert[4] installed Molteno implants into both eyes of rabbits and injected 5-FU subconjunctivally to one eye of each rabbit for 14 days postoperatively. No difference in IOPs was found at the conclusion of the eight-week study period. Prata and colleagues[5] installed 200 mm² Baerveldt implants in both eyes of rabbits, applying MMC around the equatorial explant intraoperatively in one eye of each rabbit. The MMC-treated eyes had lower IOPs initially, but no difference in IOPs was noted after week 10 to the conclusion of the study at 24 weeks; wound leaks and dehiscence occurred only in the MMC eyes. This study suggested that MMC had the potential to favorably affect the short-term clinical results of aqueous shunting surgery; however potential hazards of MMC were also observed.

Krupin and colleagues[6] conducted a prospective clinical trial with and without intraoperative MMC during the installation of single-plate Molteno implants, finding no significant difference in IOPs between the two groups at 18 months. Lee and colleagues[7] had similar IOP findings; however early hypotony occurred more often in the MMC eyes. Furthermore, Susanna and colleagues[8] experienced a high rate of explant erosion through the conjunctiva after MMC; in those eyes, conjunctival repair failed and implant removal was required.

In contrast, Perkins and colleagues[9] obtained favorable results with double-plate Molteno implantations with intraoperative MMC compared to historical controls. Significantly more MMC-treated eyes achieved IOPs in the lower teens than control eyes. However, an increased rate of early hypotony was observed in the MMC-treated eyes, so the authors suggested waiting until six weeks postoperatively before opening the ligated tube rather than their usual two weeks. In a subsequent, masked, randomized, prospective clinical study, Cantor and coauthors[10] were not able to duplicate the favorable results of Perkins and colleagues. Perhaps influencing their findings, Cantor and coauthors used a lower MMC concentration and shorter MMC exposure time compared to the former report. Nonetheless, except at week 1 when IOPs were significantly lower among MMC-treated eyes, they found no difference in IOPs through 1 year. Recently, Costa and colleagues[11] observed no significant difference in IOP reduction in a prospective randomized clinical trial of the Ahmed implant with and without intraoperative application of MMC.

In summary, some investigators have advocated MMC use with aqueous shunting surgery, but its benefit has not been confirmed by most reports. Because the role of MMC or 5-FU in aqueous shunting surgery has not been well defined and many studies have suggested higher complications rates at least with the former, the authors do not favor their use. Future studies are needed to more clearly delineate their role in aqueous shunting procedures.

REFERENCES

1. Heuer DK, Lloyd MA, Abrams DA, et al. Which is better? One or two? A randomized clinical trial of single-plate versus double-plate Molteno implantation for glaucomas in aphakia and pseudophakia. Ophthalmology, 1992;99:1512.

2. Lloyd M, Baerveldt G, Fellenbaum P, et al. Intermediate-term results of a randomized clinical trial of the 350- versus 500-mm² Baerveldt implant. Ophthalmology, 1994; 101:1456.

3. Classen L, Divella T, Tarkkenan A. Histopathologic and immunological analysis of the filtration bleb after unsuccessful glaucoma seton implantation. Am J Ophthalmol, 1996; 122:205.

4. Michel JW, Egbert PR. The effect of 5-fluorouracil on Molteno implants in rabbits [Abstracts]. Invest Ophthalmol Vis Sci, 1992;33(suppl):1272.

5. Prata JA, Minckler DS, Mermoud A, et al. Effects of intraoperative mitomycin-C on the function of Baerveldt glaucoma drainage implants in rabbits. J Glaucoma, 1996; 5:29-38.

6. Krupin TH, Birt CM, Shin DH, et al. Long term outcome of Molteno device implantation with or without adjunctive mitomycin-C use [Abstract]. Invest Ophthalmol, 1994; 35:1915.

7. Lee D, Shin D, Birt C, et al. The effect of adjunctive mitomycin C in Molteno implant surgery. Ophthalmology, 1997;104:2126-2135.

8. Susanna RJ, Nicolela M, Takahashi W. Mitomycin C as adjunctive therapy with glaucoma implant surgery. Ophthalmic Surg, 1994;25:458.

9. Perkins TW, Cardakli UF, Eisele JR, et al. Adjunctive mitomycin C in Molteno implant surgery. Ophthalmology, 1995;101:91-97.

10. Cantor L, Burgoyne J, Sanders S, et al. The effect of mitomycin C on Molteno implant surgery: A 1-year randomized, masked, prospective study. J Glaucoma, 1998; 7:240-246.

11. Costa VP, Azuara-Blanco A, Netland PA, et al. Efficacy and Safety of Adjunctive Mitomycin C during Ahmed Valve Implantation. Ophthalmology 2004;111:1071-1076.

Question 62

What are the main complications of glaucoma implant surgery?

Felix Gil Carrasco

The most frequent complications after implant surgery are not related to the surgeon. However the ones that can produce permanent damage are related to the surgeon's skills, diagnosis, anesthesia and selection of the operative technique.

There are immediate and late complications depending on whether they occur before or after the first postoperative month.

After any implant we commonly see shallow anterior chambers and hypotony due to choroidal detachments within the first two weeks after surgery.

Most of the cases respond well to the use of cyclopegics and steroids (at high doses).

Surgical drainage and anterior chamber reformation with high density viscoelastic material are only required in cases with prolonged hypotony to prevent corneal decompensation and cataract formation. In cases with flat anterior chamber and hypertension, pupillary and/or ciliary block glaucoma or hemorrhagic choroidal detachment should be suspected. The treatment in these cases is conventional. The prophylactic use of cyclopegics in the postoperative period may reduce these complications.

Hyphema may be common in cases with Neovascular Glaucoma or with peripheral anterior synechiae. In these cases introduction of the tube into the anterior chamber should be done closer to the cornea to avoid the neovascularization. If a blood clot occludes the tube, hypertension should be treated with topical medication . An attempt can be made to lyse You can try to cut the clot with a YAG-laser directed towards the tip of the tube after 72 hours, but in some cases it is necessary to washout the anterior chamber and reform it with high density viscoelastic material to stop the bleeding vessel.

Complications caused by inadequate position or length of the tube inside the anterior chamber are more common when the surgeon does not have a lot of experience. Tubes that are too close to the cornea or lens may produce decompensation of these structures and require surgical relocation.

Encapsulation of the filtering bleb with ocular hypertension constitutes the main complication after implant surgery and usually occurs two weeks after surgery. Treatment is controversial, some authors recommend an early massage to obtain an increase in the size of the filtering area and others recommend discission of the walls of the cyst when you want to preserve the implant and lower the intraocular pressure. We call this procedure "unroofing".

This must be done four months after surgery, because the "earlier the unroofing, the earlier the new encapsulation".

Other uncommon complications are tube and/or plate exposure. Although these complications are usually due to an inadequate technique, it is convenient to highlight the importance of the quality and conditions of the tissue to select the proper quadrant. With exposure of the tube or plate, the implant should be removed and replaced by a new one.

MAIN COMPLICATIONS IN DRAINAGE DEVICES

Serous Choroidal Detachment
Flat or Shallow Anterior Chamber
Hypotony
Encapsulated Bleb
Hyphema or Clot
Cataract Persistent Hypotony
Corneal Decompensation
Tube or Plate Exposure

REFERENCES

1. Melamed et al. : Postoperative complications after Molteno Implant Surgery. Am Journal Ophthalmol, 1991;111:319-22.

2. Siegner et al.: Clinical Experience with fue Baerveldt Glaucoma Drainage Implant Ophthalmol, 102:1298-1307.

3. F-ellenbaum et al.: Krupin Disk Implantation forro complicated glaucomas. Ophthalmol, 1994;101: 1178-1182.

4. Ayyala, R S., et al.: A clinical study ofthe Ahmed Glaucoma Valve Implant in Advanced Glaucoma. Ophthalmol, 1998;105: 1968-1976.

5. Lloyd M. A. et al.: Intermediate term results of a Randomized clinical trial of the 350 vs 500 mm Baerveldth Implant. Ophthalmol, 1994;101:1456-1464.

6. Gil-Carrasco, F. et al.: Ahmed valve implant for uncontolled uveitic glaucoma. Ocular Immunology and Inflammation, 1998;6:27-37.

7. Englert, J. et al.: The Ahmed Valve in Refractory Pediatric Glaucoma. Am J Ophthalmol, 1999; 127:34-42.

8. Heuer, D.K, et al.: Which is Better? One or two? A randomized clinical trial of single-plate vs double plate Molteno implantation for glaucomas in aphakia and pseudophakia. Ophthalmol, 1992; 99:1512-19.

9. Gil-Carrasco, F, et al.:Complications following Ahmed Valve implantation for uncontrolled glaucoma. Ophthalmol, (suppl)103:135. 1996.

Question 63

What are the indications for laser cyclodestructive procedures?

Jonathan G. Crowston

A number of lasers have been used to perform trans-scleral cyclodestruction since Beckman and Sugar popularized the ruby laser in the early 1970's.[1] More recently, the semiconductor diode laser has become the instrument of choice. and will provide the focus for this article.

This 810nm solid-state laser is selectively absorbed by melanin in the ciliary body permitting the use of lower laser energy compared to the Nd-YAG laser. The diode laser is compact and portable. Treatment is quick, simple and can be performed in the office environment under local anesthesia. Laser is most commonly applied trans-sclerally with a G-probe, but can also be applied endoscopically with a 21-gauge ocular endoscope inserted through the limbus or pars plana.[2] This has the advantage of permitting direct visualization of the ciliary body, but carries many of the risks associated with an intraocular surgical procedure. Although sight threatening complications appear to be less frequent compared to other cyclodestructive procedures or seton implant surgery, a number of case reports have documented the occurrence of phthisis, panuveitis, sympathetic uveitis, malignant glaucoma and hypotony maculopathy.

Traditional indications for DLCP have been restricted to painful eyes with poor visual potential or refractory glaucomas resistant to other treatments.[3] Other conditions commonly treated with DLCP include neovascular glaucoma, aphakic eyes, traumatic glaucoma, advanced developmental glaucomas as well as silicone oil-induced glaucoma or glaucoma following penetrating keratoplasty. Treatment success, usually defined in terms of IOP reduction, is fairly consistent between studies despite differences in the definition of success and the methodologies used (Table 1). The small

291

Table 1. Summary of outcomes of cyclodiode laser cylcophotocoagulation (NA=mot available)

Author/date	Number of eyes	Design	Diagnoses	Mean follow up	Definition of success	%Success	Mean number of treatments	Treatment parameters	Mean Preop IOP (mmHg)	Mean Post Op IOP (mmHg)
Schlote (2001)[4]	93	Prospective non comparative interventional case series	Refractory (mixed aetiology)	12 months	Final IOP >5<21mmHg	74%	1.9	10 to 15 x 2.0W x 1.5 to 2s	42.1=/-11.0	17.3=/-10.9
Bloom (1997)[5]	210	Non comparative interventional case series	Refractory (mixed aetiology)	10 months	<22mmHg <17mmHg 30% reduction	66%	1.75	90J 120J (re-treatment)	34.1+/-10.6	20.1+/-9.3
Kirwan (2002)[6]	77	Non comparative interventional case series	Refractory (paediatric)	21 months	<22mmHg or 30% reduction	72% (1-year) 51% (2-years)	2.3	40 x 1.5W x 1.5s	32.0+/-6.4	22.5+/9.7
Spencer (1999)[7]	58	Non comparative interventional case series	Refractory (mixed aetiology)	18.7 months	<22mmHg <17mmHg 30% reduction	81% 59% 78%	1.6	14 x 2.0W x 2 s	33.0+/- 10.7	16.7 +/7.8
Egbert (2001)[8]	92	Prospective	Primary open angle glaucoma	13.2 months	>20%	47%	1	20 x 1.5W x 1.5s or 1.25W x 2.5s	29+/-8.9	25.7+/-10.3
Mistlberger (2001)[9]	206	Non comparative interventional case series	Refractory (mixed aetiology)	9.2 months	<22mmHg	66.9% (1-year) 49.85% (2-year)	NA	19 x 1.75W x 2s	42.1+/-11.0	17.3+/-10.9
Lai (2003)[10]	14	Prospective non comparative	Chronic angle closure glaucoma	12 months	NA	NA	1.1	16 x 2W x 2s	36.9+/-11.7	18.9+/-6.5
Lima (2004)[12]	68	Prospective alternating (Endoscopic cyclophotocoagulation vs Ahmed Implant)	Refractory (mixed aetiology)	24 months	>6mmHg <21mmHg	74% ECP 71% AI	1	0.5W x 2s (210°)	41.6+/-3.2	14.1+/-7.2

numbers of patients in these studies limits the usefulness of subgroup analysis regarding outcomes in the different types of glaucoma. This in mind, it appears that DLCP generally has a higher success rate with neovascular, uveitic and primary open angle glaucoma generally have a higher success rate than with aphakic, traumatic or paediatric glaucomas.[4]

A wider scope for DLPC has been predicted, as experience of the long-term outcomes of treatment grows.[4,5] A number of reports document the use of DLCP in eyes with advanced glaucoma that have not undergone previous incisional surgery. This may be appropriate in cases such as neovascular glaucoma which carry a poor prognosis with trabeculectomy or seton implant surgery [5] In some centers, DLCP has largely replaced seton implant surgery as the treatment of choice . A more controversial role is the use of DLPC as a primary surgical therapy for advanced glaucoma in developing countries where access to other treatments are limited by financial and logistic restraints. In a prospective study of West Africans with advanced POAG, IOP lowering was only modest with only 47% achieving a 20% reduction in IOP after a single application.[6] This suggests that IOP lowering in this population of patients is not sufficient with cyclodiode alone.

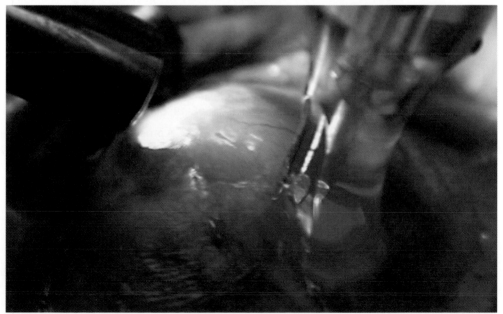

Figure 1. G-probe of the diode laser is positioned over the ciliary body identified as a dark band by transillumination. (courtesy of Dr Tony Wells and www.eyetext.net)

Based on current evidence, the American Academy of Ophthalmology has recommended that DLCP is indicated for patients with refractory glaucoma who have failed trabeculectomy or seton tube implant surgery, patients with elevated IOP and limited visual potential and also for pain relief in eyes with no visual potential. Cyclophotocoagulation may also have a useful role for patients with acute onset neovascular glaucoma, or in patients whose general medical condition precludes more invasive surgery or where the risks of such surgery are large. Further evidence derived from prospective randomised clinical trials comparing DLCP with antimetabolite-augmented trabeculectomy or seton implant surgery are required to properly evaluate this treatment.

REFERENCES

1. Beckman H, Kinoshita A, Rota AN, Sugar HS. Transscleral ruby laser irradiation of the ciliary body in the treatment of intractable glaucoma. Trans Am Acad Ophthalmol Otolaryngol,. 1972;76:423-36.

2. Uram M. Endoscopic cyclophotocoagulation in glaucoma management. Curr Opin Ophthalmol, 1995;6:19-29.

3. Martin KR, Broadway DC. Cyclodiode laser therapy for painful, blind glaucomatous eyes. Br J Ophthalmol,. 2001;85:474-6.

4. Schlote T, Derse M, Rassmann K, Nicaeus T, Dietz K, Thiel HJ. Efficacy and safety of contact transscleral diode laser cyclophotocoagulation for advanced glaucoma. J Glaucoma, 2001;10:294-301.

5. Bloom PA, Tsai JC, Sharma K, Miller MH, Rice NS, Hitchings RA, Khaw PT. "Cyclodiode". Trans-scleral diode laser cyclophotocoagulation in the treatment of advanced refractory glaucoma. Ophthalmology,. 1997;104:1508-19; discussion 1519-20.

6. Egbert PR, Williams AS, Singh K, Dadzie P, Egbert TB. A prospective trial of intraoperative fluorouracil during trabeculectomy in a black population. Am J Ophthalmol, 1993;116:612-6.

7. Kirwan JF, Shah P, Khaw PT. Diode laser cyclophotocoagulation: role in the management of refractory pediatric glaucomas. Ophthalmology, 2002;109:316-23.

8. Spencer AF, Vernon SA. "Cyclodiode": results of a standard protocol. Br J Ophthalmol, 1999;83:311-6.

9. Egbert PR, Fiadoyor S, Budenz DL, Dadzie P, Byrd S. Diode laser transscleral cyclophotocoagulation as a primary surgical treatment for primary open-angle glaucoma. Arch Ophthalmol, 2001;119:345-50.

10. Mistlberger A, Liebmann JM, Tschiderer H, Ritch R, Ruckhofer J, Grabner G. Diode laser transscleral cyclophotocoagulation for refractory glaucoma. J Glaucoma, 2001;10:288-93.

11. Lai JS, Tham CC, Chan JC, Lam DS. Diode laser transscleral cyclophotocoagulation in the treatment of chronic angle-closure glaucoma: a preliminary study. J Glaucoma, 2003;12:360-4.

12. Lima FE, Magacho L, Carvalho DM, Susanna R, Jr., Avila MP. A prospective, comparative study between endoscopic cyclophotocoagulation and the Ahmed drainage implant in refractory glaucoma. J Glaucoma, 2004;13:233-7.

Index

Page numbers in *italic* are reffered *table*.

C

Cataract
   and glaucoma, 269-273
      combined procedures, 269-273
         indications for, 269-273
      sequential management of, 269
      combined surgery, 271
         indications for, 271
      summary, 273
   removal, 270
      alone, 270
      via temporal, 270
      in an eye, 271
Cataract Persistent Hypotomy, *288*
Chronic Angle Closure
   management in, 185-186
      patient with, 185-186
Choroidal Effusion
   after trabeculectomy, 251-252
Chronic Glaucoma, 262
Chronic Uveitis, 263
Ciliary Block, 177
Clot, Hyphema or, *288*
Color Vision
   loss of, 89
Compressive Optic Neuropathy, *90*
Conjunctival Clamp, 231
   explanation, 231
Conjunctival Closure, 233
Conjunctival Inflammatory Disease, 262
Corneal Decompensation, *288*
Corneal Epithelial Defects, 225
Cup/Disc Ratios, 42
CYP1B1
   disease, *37*

D

Deep Sclerectomy, 275
Drug(s)
   ideal characteristcs of, 91-93
      for the treatment, 91-93

E

Early glaucoma
   treatment of, 135-139
      IOP reduction effective, 135
      the goal of, 136
      natural history, 136
      velocity of progression, 136
      early treatment, 136
      intial treatment, 136
      course of the disease, 139
      summary, 139
Egbert, Study
   number of eyes, *292*
   design, *292*
   diagnoses, *292*
   mean follow up, *292*
   definition of success, *292*
   % success, *292*
   number of treatment, *292*
   treatment parameters, *292*
   mean preop IOP, *292*
   mean post Op IOP, *292*
Egna-Neumarkt Eye Study[20], *5*
Encapsulated Bleb, *288*
Exfoliation Syndrome, *37*
   control in, 157-160
      IOP difficult to, 157-160

F

Failing Bleb
diagnose, 261-264
management, 261-264
conditions under 1, 263
conditions under 2, 263
"successful" bleb, 261
development of the, 261
FDT
in clinical evaluation, 67-68
of glaucoma, 67-68
5-Fluorouracil
in trabeculectomy, 221-225
in aqueous shunting procedures, 283-285
FOXC1
disease, *37*
Framingham Study[21], *5*
Frequency Doubling Technology, *see FDT*, 67-68

G

Genetic Testing, 35-37
Glaucoma
biological definition, 1
clinical definition, 2
structural changes, 2
functional changes, 3
case definition of, 3
people go blind from, 9-11
new technological application in, 9
causes blindness, 9
preventable, 10
how often do patients with, 13
single screening examinations, 13
lont-term follow-up, 14
some people go blind from, 14
selective cell death in, 21-25
experimental indicates, 23
in only eye disease, 27-33
implication, 32
chronic open angle, 27
experimental primate model, 31
genetic testing, 35-37
clinical evaluation of, 51-54, 61-74
optical coherence tomography, 51-54
scanning laser polarimetry in, 61-65
FDT perimetry in, 67-68
SWAP in, 71-74
introduction, 71
pachymetry in, 113-115
practical importance of, 113-115
evaluation of, 57-59, 77-79
introduction, 57
glaucomatous optic disc, 57
detection of, 57
progression, 58
detection of, 58
conclusion, 59
UBM in, 77-79
blood flow, 99-101
practical importance of, 99-101
diagnosis, 81-83
management, 81-85, 141-143, 201-205
progression in the, 141-143
FACT presumes, 142

299

cup/disc ratios, 42

optic disc hemorrhages, 43

parapapillary chorioretinal atrophy, 44

retinal arterioles, 46

   diameter of, 46

retinal nerve fiber layer, 47

   evaluation of the, 47

Gonioscopy, 167

H

Hyphema, 225

Hypotony, *288*

Hypotony Maculopathy, 253-256

   in overfiltration, 253-256

I

Intraocular Pressure, *see IOP*, 15

IOP, 15

   elevated, 117

     prevalence of, 117

   all levels of, 117

     glaucomatous damage at, 117

     fluctuation, 125-126

     importance of, 125-126

      in glaucoma, 125-126

   reduction effective, 135

   difficult to control, 157-160

     in exfoliation syndrome, 157-160

Iridocorneal Angle, 167

Iris Hypoplasia, *37*

J

Juvenile Open Angle Glaucoma, *37*

K

Kirwan, Study

   number of eyes, *292*

   design, *292*

   diagnoses, *292*

   mean follow up, *292*

   definition of success, *292*

   % success, *292*

   number of treatment, *292*

   treatment parameters, *292*

   mean preop IOP, *292*

   mean post Op IOP, *292*

Kjere Optic Neuropathy, *90*

L

Lai, Study

   number of eyes, *292*

   design, *292*

   diagnoses, *292*

   mean follow up, *292*

   definition of success, *292*

   % success, *292*

   number of treatment, *292*

   treatment parameters, *292*

   mean preop IOP, *292*

   mean post Op IOP, *292*

Laser Cyclodestructive Procedures

   indications for, 291-294

Laser Iridoplasty

   performed by, 213-214

   Laser Iridotomy

   in management, 153-156, 193-195

     of PDS, 153-156

     of PACG, 193

      limitations of, 193-195

Myocilin
    disease, *37*
Myopic Eyes
    and glaucomatous damage, 117-119

N

Nanophthalmia, 189
Nanophthalmic Eyes
    glaucoma in, 189-191
        diagnose, 189-191
        manage, 189-191
Neovascular Glaucoma
    effectively managed, 163-165
Neuroretinal Rim Pallor, 41
Neuroretinal Rim Shape, 41
Neuroretinal Rim Size, 40
Non Penetrating Surgery
    indications for, 275-277
        deep sclerectomy, 275
        viscocanalostomy, 276
Normal Tension Glaucoma, *37*

O

Occludable Angle
    detection of, 171-173
    management of, 171-172
OCT, 51-54
Ocular Blood Flow
    methods for assessing, 81-83
Ocular Hypertension, *37*
Ocular Hypertension Treatment Study, *see OHTS*, 109
Ocular Hypertensives, 109-110
Ocular Trauma, 79
OHTS, 109
OPA1

disease, *37*
Optical Coherence Tomography, *see OCT*, 51-54
Optic Cup Size, 42
Optic Disc Hemorrhages, 43
Optic Disc Size, 40
Optic Nerve Damage
    causes of, 17-19
        in glaucoma, 17-19
Optic Neuropathy, 17
Optineurin
    disease, *37*
Overfiltration
    hypotomy maculopathy due to, 253-256

P

PAC, 171
PACG, 171, 175-178
    forces causing, 175
    definitive treatment, 175
    management of, 193-195
        laser iridotomy in the, 193-195
            limitations of, 193-195
Pachymetry
    practical importance of, 113-115
        in the clinical evaluation, 113-115
        of glaucoma, 113-115
Parapapillary Chorioretinal Atrophy, 44
PAX6
    disease, *37*
PDS
    management of, 153-156
        laser iridotomy in the, 153-156
Pediatric Glaucoma, 279
Persistent Choroidal Effusions, 224